LOVE YOUR HAIR

LOOK BOOK

Real Women. Real Beauty. Real Stories.

by Chanel E. Martin

Copyright Page

Copyright © 2025 by Chanel E Martin All rights reserved Published by Beyondthebookmedia.com

All rights reserved. No part of this publication may be reproduced, distributed, or transmitted in any form or by any means, including photocopying, recording, or other electronic or mechanical methods, without the prior written permission of the publisher, except in the case of brief quotations embodied in critical reviews and certain other noncommercial uses permitted by copyright law. For permissionrequests, write to the publisher, addressed "Attention: Permissions Coordinator" at the address below.

Limit of Liability/Disclaimer of Warranty: While the publisher and author have used their best efforts in preparing this book, they make no representations of warranties with respect to the accuracy or completeness of the contents of this book and specifically disclaim any implied warranties or merchantability or fitness for a particular purpose. No warranty may be created or extended by sales representatives or written sales materials. The advice and strategies contained herein may not be suitable for your situation. You should consult with a professional where appropriate. Neither the publisher nor the author shall be liable for damages arising herefrom.

Beyond The Book Media, LLC
Atlanta GA
www.beyondthebookmedia.com

The publisher is not responsible for websites that are not owned by the publisher.

Love Your Hair Look Book: Real Women. Real Beauty. Real Stories.	1
Copyright Page	2
Introduction	4
About Refreshed Hair & Scalp Oil	5
Ellie Shoulders	6
Jesica Williams,	7
Kimberly Fisher	8
Marshana Green-Rostagno	9
Pain of the Press and Curl	10
La'Tasha Givens	11
Monique Davis	12
Ezinne Orji	13
Ponytail Gate	14
Morgan Makail	15
Ileisha Honeycutt	16
Te'Etta Ruth	17
My Doll Beauty Salon	18
Dr. Shannette Bone	19
Silver Moran-Stewart	20
Crystal R. Durham	21
Bobbing and Boys	22
Sarah Noelsaint	23
Cree Grier	24
Dejah Janae	25
Kool-Aid Color	26
Barbara Mukonyo	27
Destiny Thomas	28
Christal Jordan Jennings	29
Micro Braids and Microwaves	30
Kennedy Simone	31
Tiffany B. Livingston	32
Jade Nadaree	33
Lindsey A. Walker,	34
Will Work for Hair	35
Karyse J. Gocoul	36
Shiann Graneau	37
Chanel E. Martin	38

INTRODUCTION

I love hair and beauty. It was the whole reason I became a chemical engineer. The thought of creating products and tools that help men and women look and feel their best excited me from an early age. I wanted to use my natural knack for science to help change the hair and beauty industry, not just with innovation but with intention.

By the grace of God, I've had the opportunity to do just that. As a cofounder of Myavana, one of the most innovative hair technology companies in the world, I helped develop a patented AI process that assists women in selecting the right products and services to meet their unique hair goals. During our early research and development, I spent countless hours examining strands of hair under a high-powered microscope. It was in those moments that I truly began to understand the science of hair health—and how deeply it connects to our confidence, our identity, and even our self-worth.

My mission has always been simple: to help women love the hair God gave them and embrace their unique hair journeys, no matter the texture, length, or story behind it. That mission is what led me to develop Refreshed Hair & Scalp Oil, a proprietary blend of vitamins and essential oils designed to help women experience real hair growth in just 30 to 90 days.

Through my research and personal experiences, I discovered that hair growth is more than just about the products we use; it's also about how we care for ourselves. Scalp health, wellness, nutrition, and movement all play a role. That's why I launched the Grow Your Hair Challenge, combining physical fitness, nutrition, mindset, and a simple hair care regimen to support women with busy lifestyles. (You can check it out at growyourhairchallenge.com.)

Now, with the Love Your Hair Lookbook, my heart is to celebrate beauty in all its forms—to showcase real women across different skin tones, hair types, and textures and to amplify what they love about their hair. I also share a few personal stories sprinkled in between, along with photos of my many hairstyles over the years! My prayer is that you find these stories relatable and fun!

Hair, especially for Black women, has too often been stigmatized or politicized. But our hair is sacred. It is powerful. It is personal. It carries stories, history, resilience, and expression. And that is why we must love our hair, with intention, with pride, and without apology.

I hope you use this Lookbook as more than a visual guide. Let it be a conversation starter. A reason to pause and affirm the beauty within yourself and in others. Share it. Talk about it. Celebrate it.

Because when we love our hair, we're really loving ourselves. And that is always worth honoring.

Chanel E. Martin

Founder, Her Beauty Regimen

ABOUT REFRESHED HAIR & SCALP OIL

When I created Refreshed Hair & Scalp Oil, I wasn't trying to follow a trend or fill a shelf—I was solving a problem I knew intimately. I had lost my hair not once, but multiple times. After childbirth. After stress. After years of protective styling and product buildup. I know the pain of watching your hair thin, break off, or simply not thrive the way it should. I also know what it feels like to search endlessly for something that works—not just for growth but for true restoration.

As a chemical engineer, I understand how ingredients work—not just how they sound in marketing but what they actually do for your scalp and hair strands on a cellular level. That's the foundation I used to formulate Refreshed Hair & Scalp Oil: a lightweight, non-greasy, deeply nourishing blend of 11 premium oils, hand-selected for their ability to support growth, reduce inflammation, and maintain moisture at the root—without clogging the pores or causing buildup.

This isn't just another oil in a pretty bottle. Refreshed was created with intention, backed by science, and tested by real women with real results. It's especially formulated for women who wear protective styles, wigs, weaves, or locs—women who are often overlooked in mainstream haircare conversations. Your scalp matters, even when your hair is tucked away. Without a healthy scalp, growth will always be limited.

What Makes Refreshed Different?

- Lightweight Formula: Absorbs quickly without leaving residue or buildup
- 11-Nutrient Blend: Including ingredients like castor oil, jojoba, peppermint, rosemary, tea tree, and more—each selected for its regenerative, antimicrobial, or anti-inflammatory properties
- Promotes Growth in 30–90 Days: When used consistently as part of a healthy regimen, users have reported noticeable thickening, length retention, and stronger roots
- Soothes the Scalp: Helps reduce flaking, itchiness, and inflammation, creating the right environment for growth
- Versatile Application: Can be used on the scalp, edges, or as a hot oil treatment before shampooing

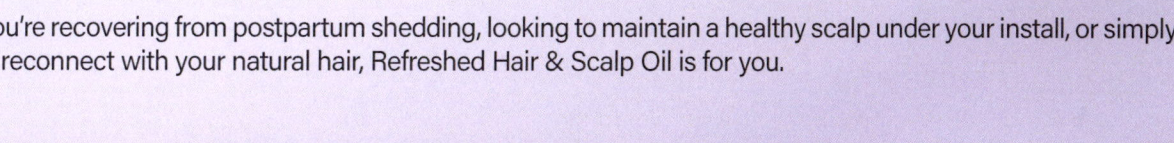

But more than what's in the bottle, Refreshed is a movement. It's a reminder that healing is possible. That your hair can grow again. That it's never too late to start over. I've watched so many women—myself included—go from discouragement to joy simply by creating space in their routines for real, intentional care.

And that's what Her Beauty Regimen is all about: giving women access to products, education, and encouragement to take their beauty journey into their own hands—with tools that actually work.

Whether you're recovering from postpartum shedding, looking to maintain a healthy scalp under your install, or simply wanting to reconnect with your natural hair, Refreshed Hair & Scalp Oil is for you.

Because when your scalp is cared for, your hair can thrive.
And when your hair thrives, your confidence follows. Order yours at HerBeautyRegimen.com

ELLIE SHOULDERS

SOCIAL MEDIA HANDLE:

Instagram, YouTube, and TikTok: @ecclesiiastes

ABOUT ELLIE:

Ellie Shoulders is a graduate of the University of Oklahoma, where she earned her degree in Information Science and Technology. She currently serves as an Event Specialist at the University of Central Oklahoma. In addition to her role in higher education, Ellie is a multi-talented entrepreneur and creative professional. She runs a catering business, Ellie's Cajun Kitchen, and also works as a model, actress, and online content creator. Ellie is passionate about using her gifts to support and uplift others in meaningful ways.

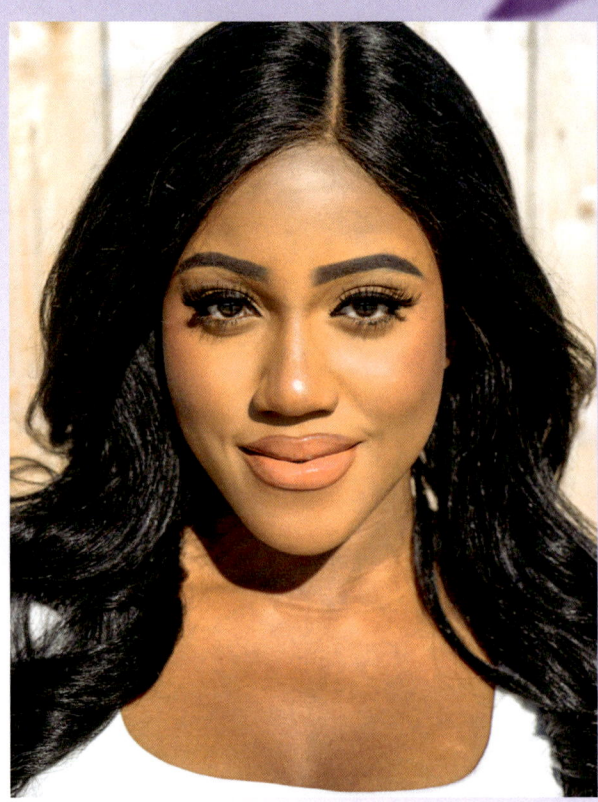

WHY DO YOU LOVE YOUR HAIR?

"I love my hair because it is a gift that my body has given me. Treat it like so."

FAVORITE BEAUTY OR HAIR HACK:

The LCO (Liquid, Cream, Oil) method for moisture retention is my tried and true method.

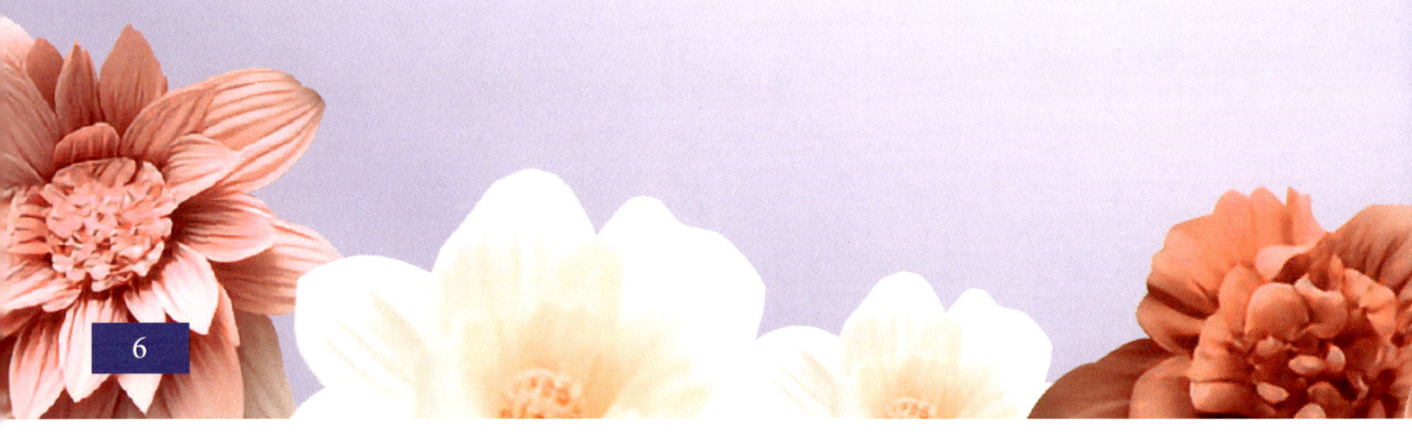

JESICA WILLIAMS

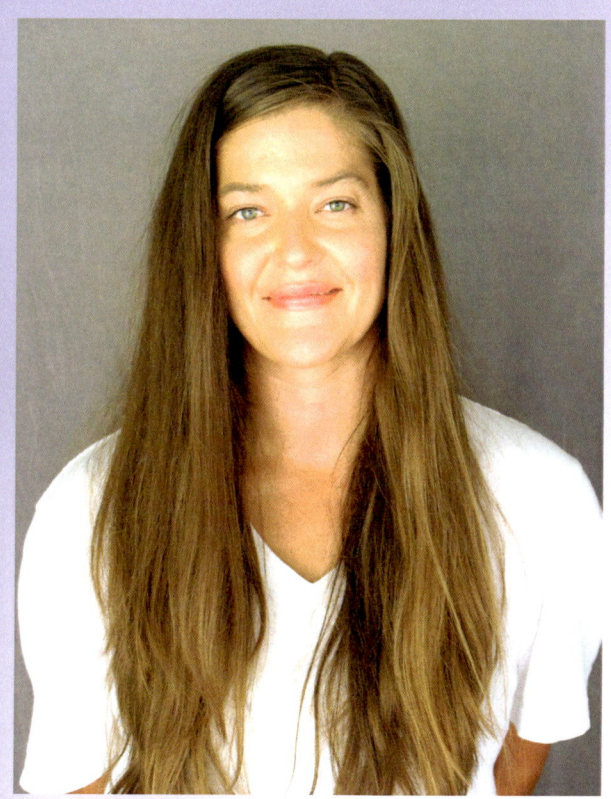

SOCIAL MEDIA HANDLE:

Instagram and TikTok: @feelmoregooder

ABOUT JESICA:

Jesica Williams is a present-day Natural Health Blogger/Researcher, crossfitter, nature seeker, and hippie. She's a former NCAA volleyball player, a lifelong athlete, and a South Florida native. Her blog is focused on healing through nature immersion (specifically sunbathing, cold plunging, and sauna therapy), and functional fitness. She lives by her mantra "make good use of your pulse" and encourages others to make their own rules in life to feel free and empowered.

WHY DO YOU LOVE YOUR HAIR?

"I love my hair because it's fully me. I don't dye it or apply any heat to it. It's frequently immersed in natural bodies of water, and I enjoy letting it be free. I've never been so happy with my hair."

FAVORITE BEAUTY OR HAIR HACK:

Wash your hair less, and ditch the chemicals.

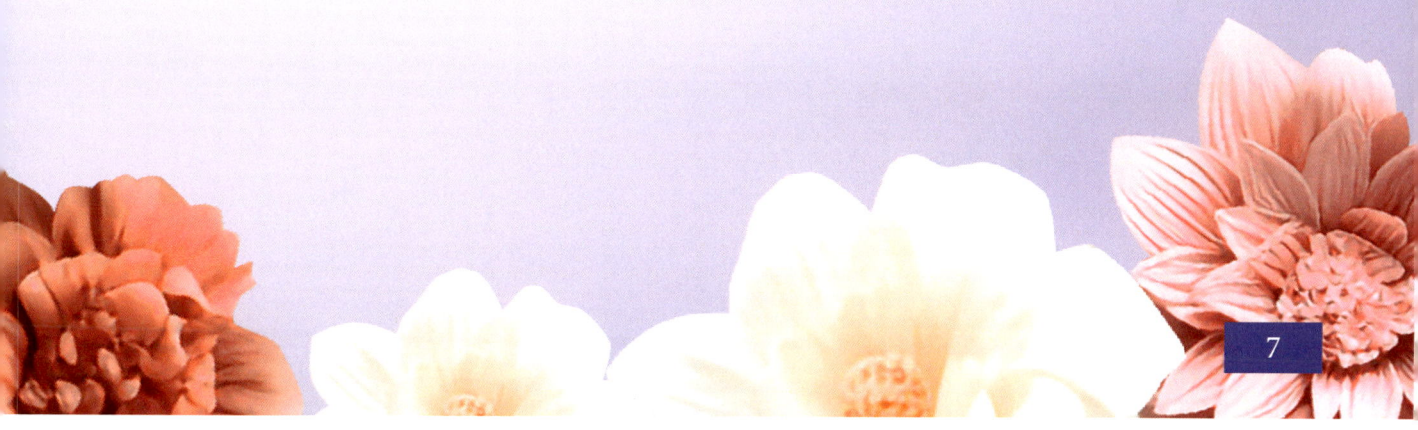

KIMBERLY FISHER

SOCIAL MEDIA HANDLE:

@itskimberlyfisher

ABOUT KIMBERLY:

Kimberly Fisher is a freelance travel writer and travel curator. She specializes in luxury travel and lifestyle and has covered art, beauty, culture, destinations, fashion, food, fitness/wellness, events, hotels, and wine & spirits.

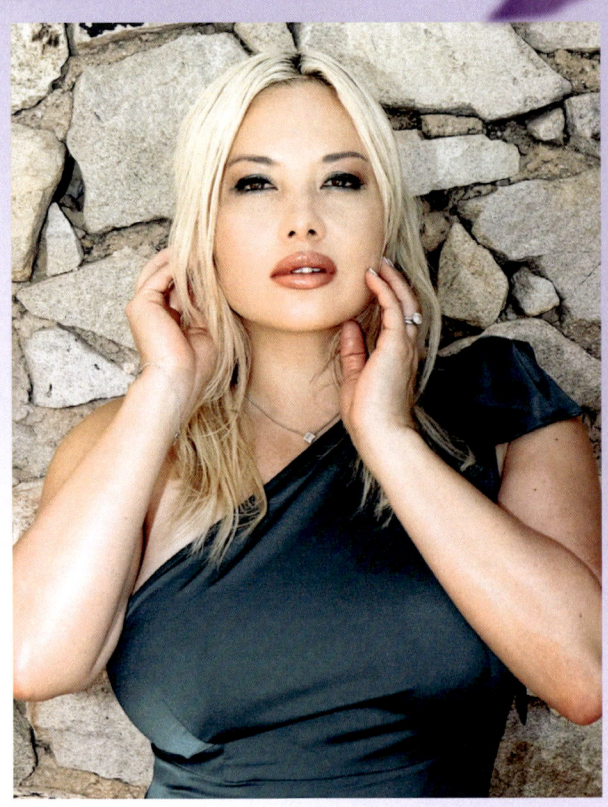

WHY DO YOU LOVE YOUR HAIR?

"I love my hair for being strong and resilient- sort of like me. :) "

FAVORITE BEAUTY OR HAIR HACK:

Heartless curlers at night and amazing serums have changed my life.

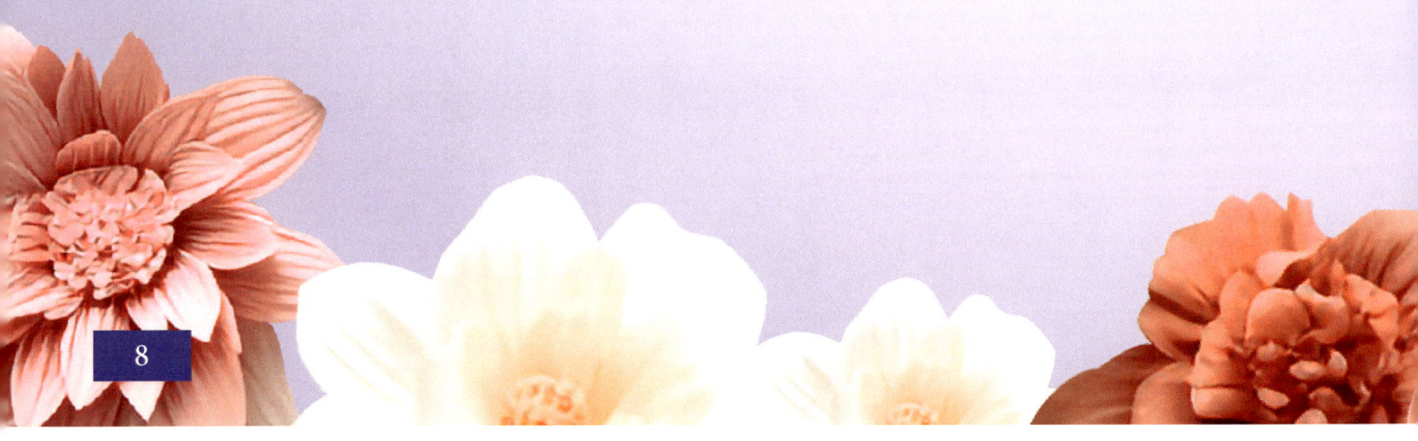

MARSHANA GREEN-ROSTAGNO

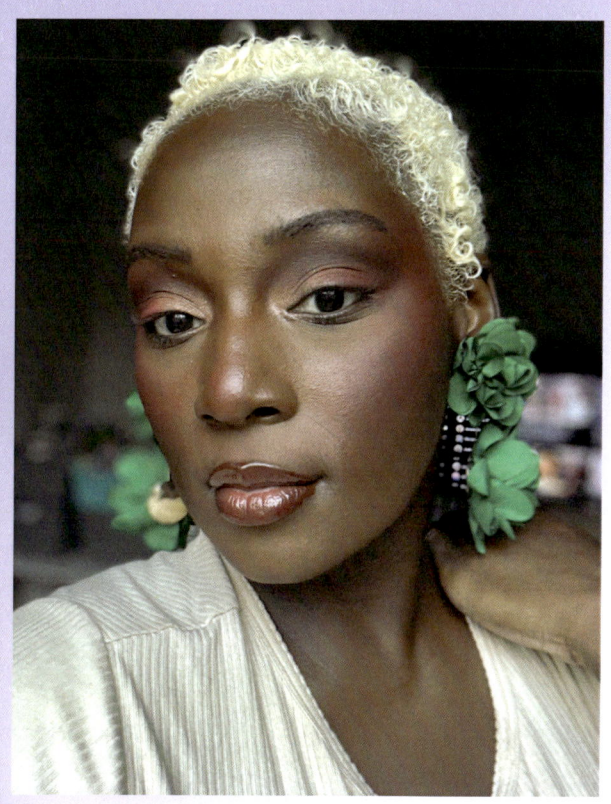

SOCIAL MEDIA HANDLE:

TikTok: the_beauty_tag
Instagram: @mgrostagno

ABOUT MARSHANA:

Marshana Green-Rostagno is passionate about beauty, fashion, hair care, and travel. She creates engaging vlogs that reflect all of these interests, offering her audience a blend of style and lifestyle content. Marshana also takes pride in supporting and spotlighting small businesses—especially Black-owned and locally owned brands—through her reviews and personal recommendations.

WHY DO YOU LOVE YOUR HAIR?

"I love my hair because it's beautiful. I would have it no other way."

FAVORITE BEAUTY OR HAIR HACK:

My favorite hair hack is a leave-in conditioner; you can use it to style, to moisturize (aside from water), and to deep condition as well! My favorite haircare product to use in under 10 minutes!

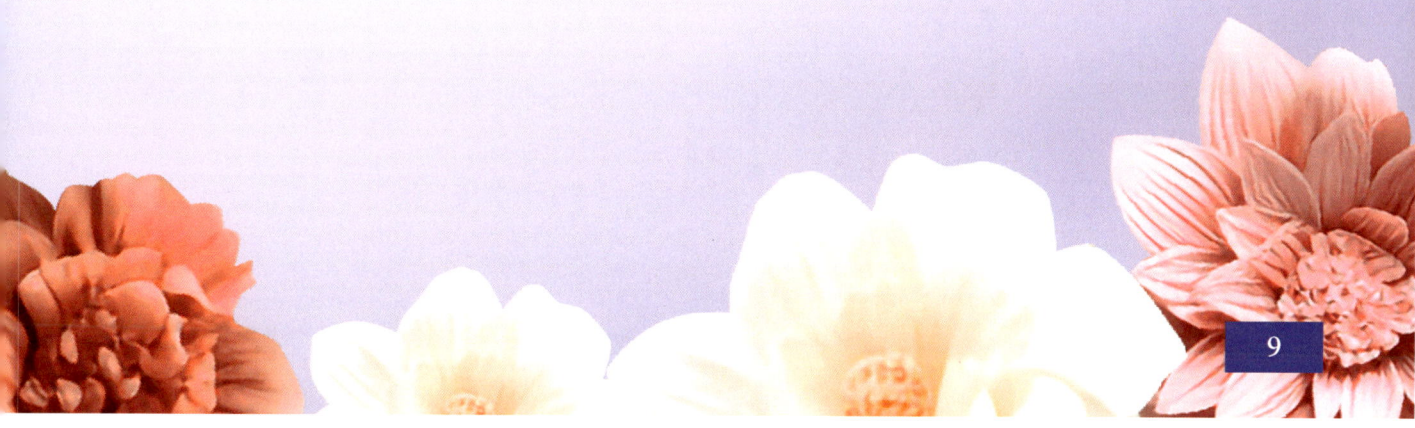

PAIN OF THE PRESS AND CURL

Growing up, like most African American little girls in the 90s, I assumed I had bad hair—mainly because all I heard was how "thick" and "nappy" my hair was. And boy, was it thick. I had a full head of kinky curly locs that cascaded down to the middle of my back. My mom, although she could do a little something-something with hair, started me out at the salon at an early age.

One of my most vivid memories was going to the beauty school in Pine Bluff, Arkansas, on the weekends while visiting my family. Early Saturday morning, my mom or aunt would book hair appointments for me and my cousins with the students. The style of choice? You guessed it—press and curl. And this might even have been before electric pressing combs were invented or accessible. My student stylist would lay the iron comb in a heating unit to heat it. She'd add a good slather of Blue Magic hair grease while I braced myself! I prayed that I wouldn't burn from the steam that sizzled off the pressing comb. I was used to the weekend ritual of press and curls. But one day, the memory turned into a nightmare.

At the young age of six years old, my hairstylist's hand slipped, and she did the unthinkable—she dropped the hot metal pressing comb on the nape of my neck. I screamed in agony, and my stylist screamed, too! She was frozen in fear, not sure what to do next. I remember the salon going into an uproar as the instructor attempted to calm me and the newly trained stylist down. The remedy was to put on a cold compress and apply burn treatment to the wound.

I bet you can imagine how upset my mother was. However, this is the risk you take when you book a student hairstylist. She did finish my hair after I calmed down, and I was Sunday School sharp! Can you believe that after all these years, I still have the burn mark on the back of my neck? I am so happy we've found safer and less scary options for straightening our hair. My daughters will never know the pain of the press and curl!

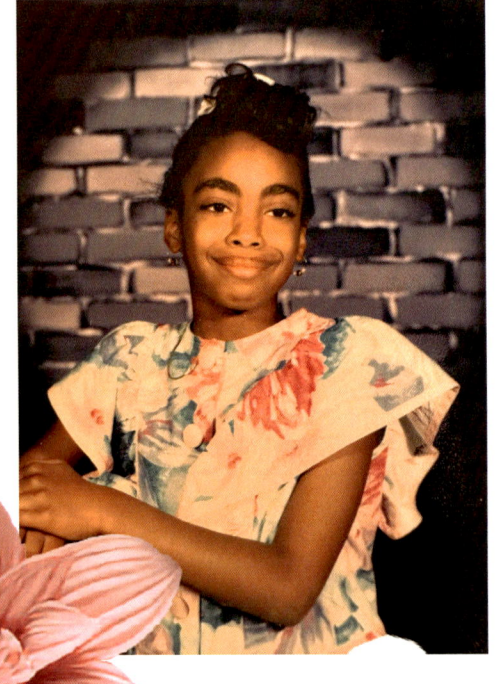

Chanel E. Martin

2nd Grade

LA'TASHA GIVENS

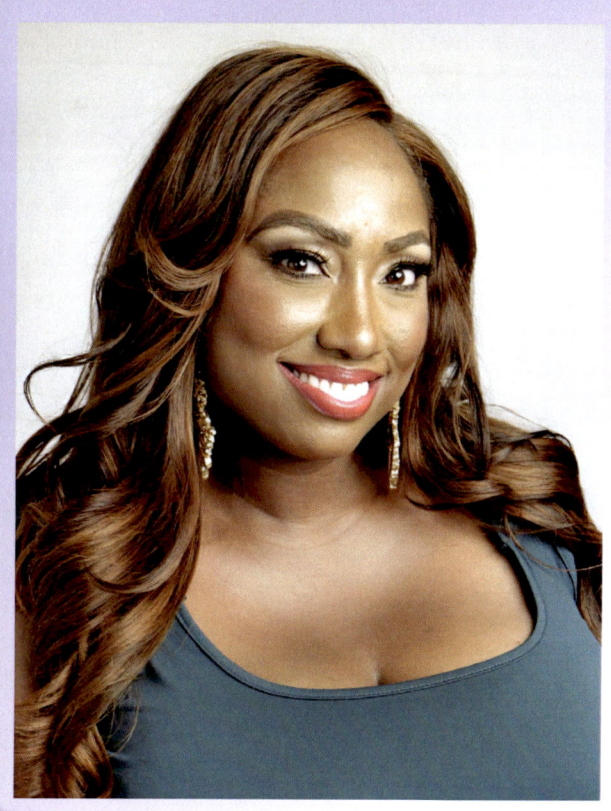

SOCIAL MEDIA HANDLE:

@latashagivens1

ABOUT LA'TASHA:

La'Tasha Givens is a two-time Emmy Award-winning reporter and anchor with nearly two decades of experience in television news, radio, and public relations. She has built a reputation as a trusted journalist, celebrated storyteller, and dedicated community advocate.

WHY DO YOU LOVE YOUR HAIR?

"I love how I can change my hair with my personality. I also love how my industry is more accepting of different hair styles for women of color."

FAVORITE BEAUTY OR HAIR HACK:

After my hair is braided for a sew-in, I completely saturate my scalp and braids with hair oil. It has changed the texture of my hair. I swear by it.

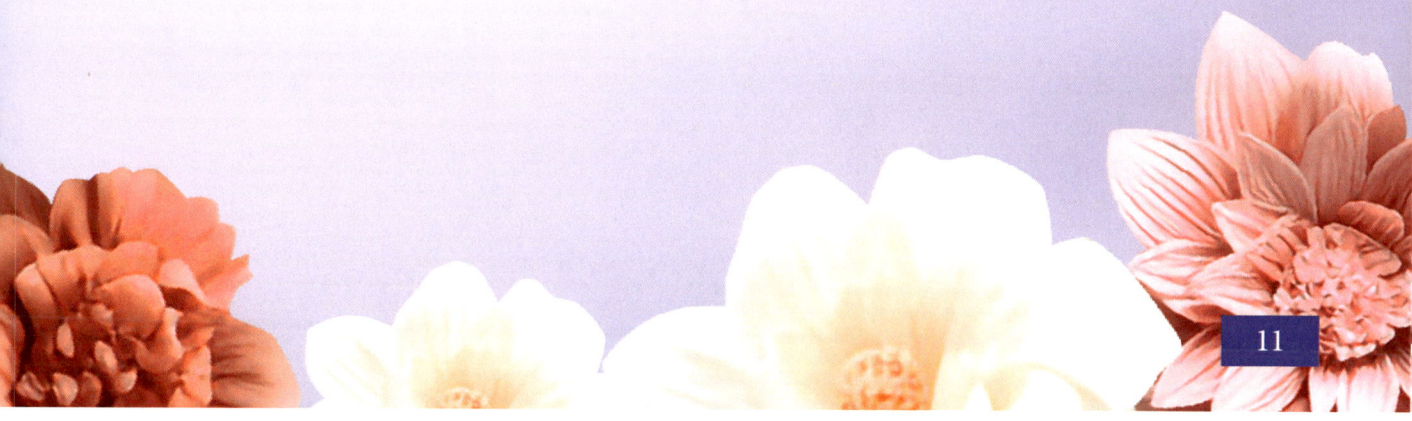

MONIQUE DAVIS
TALENT CONSULTANT & WEALTH BROKER

SOCIAL MEDIA HANDLE:

@themoniquedavis

ABOUT MONIQUE:

Monique is a multifaceted influencer, mother, and entrepreneur who seamlessly blends faith, beauty, and style. Known for her authentic presence on Amazon Live and social media, she shares her passion for hair and beauty products while inspiring women to embrace their true selves. With a background in career consulting, wealth brokerage, and community leadership, Monique brings a unique perspective to the beauty world—empowering her audience to feel confident and radiant every day.

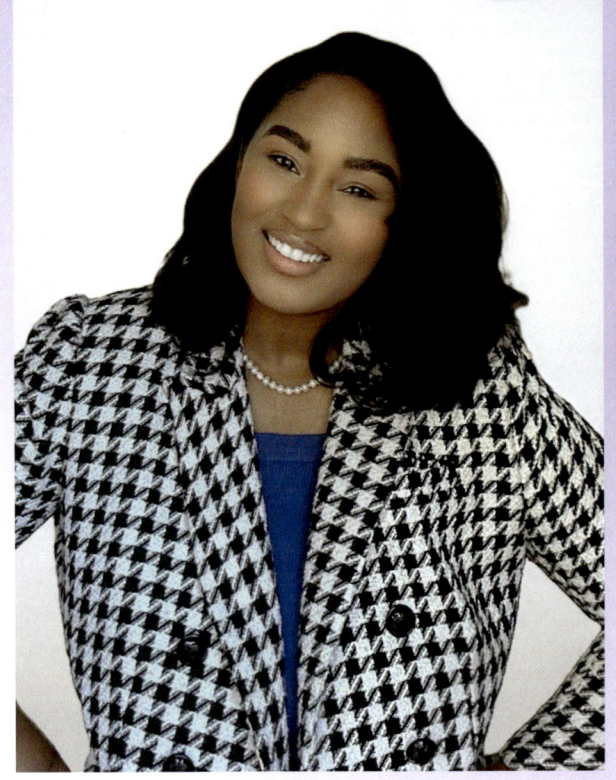

WHY DO YOU LOVE YOUR HAIR?

"I love my hair because it's a bold statement of strength, wisdom, and the rich heritage we carry. Each curl is a daily reminder of God's masterful design."

FAVORITE BEAUTY OR HAIR HACK:

I stopped shopping name brands just because they're popular. I love refreshed edge control on my edges, and it's the best I've experienced.

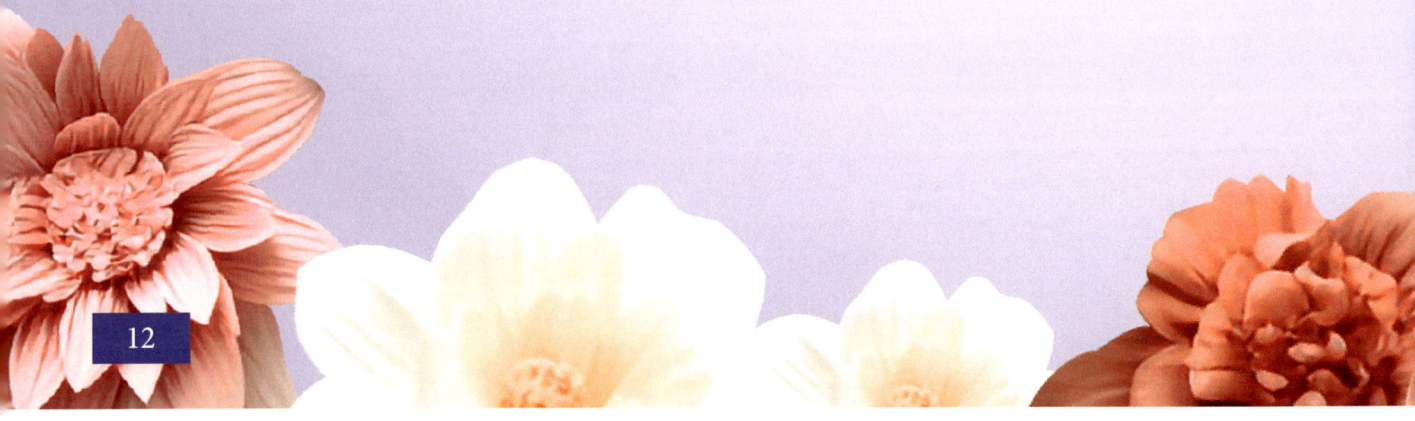

EZINNE ORJI

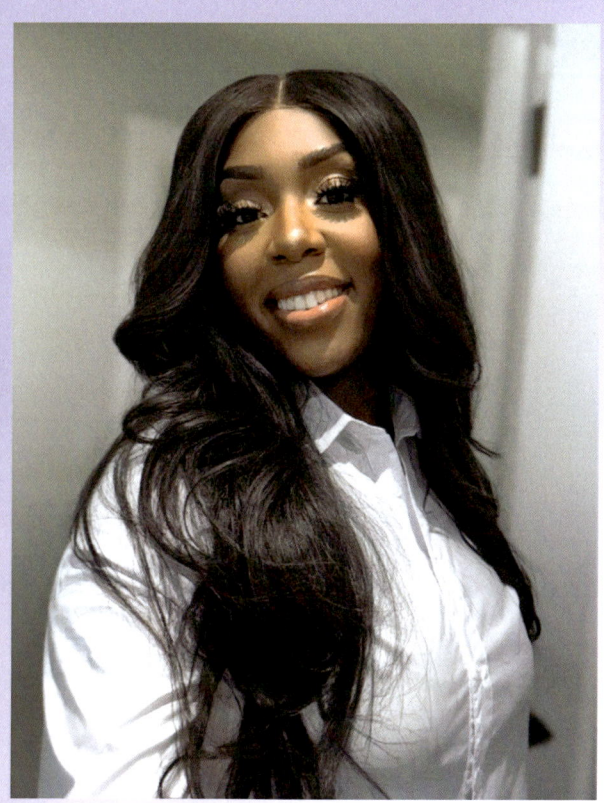

SOCIAL MEDIA HANDLE:

@ezzyyyyy_

ABOUT EZINNE:

Ezinne is a chemist and beauty enthusiast who enjoys all things related to personal care and cosmetics. She is a God-fearing wife and mother to a beautiful baby girl. She aspires to one day create her beauty brand named after her daughter.

WHY DO YOU LOVE YOUR HAIR?

"My hair is how God crowned me!"

FAVORITE BEAUTY OR HAIR HACK:

Washing my hair weekly helps my scalp breathe, and I don't have to worry about buildup.

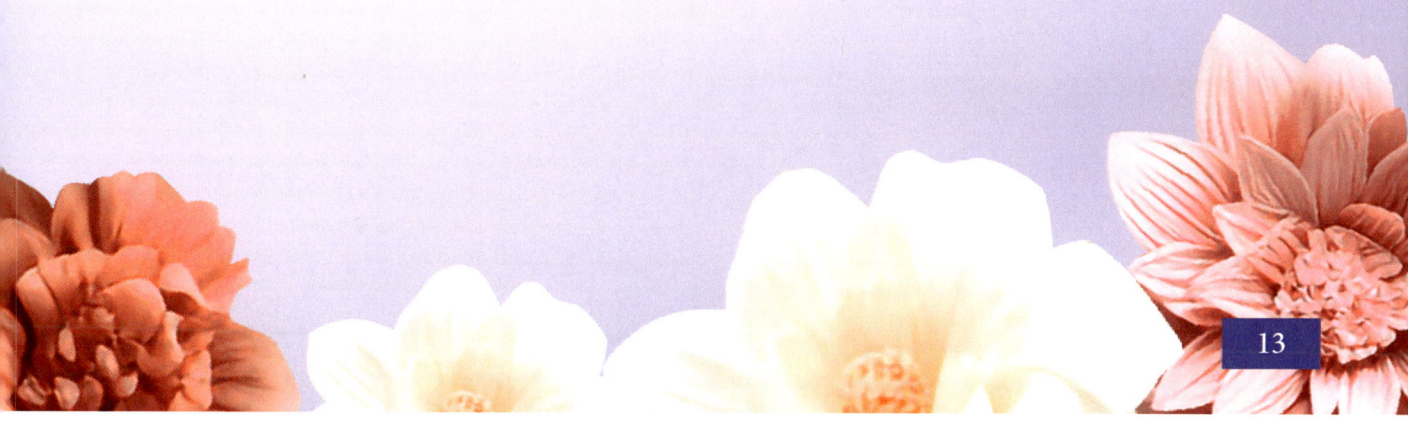

PONYTAIL GATE

My mom was a hardworking woman. When I was in the second grade, my mother worked full-time and was studying to obtain her master's degree. This often meant we had to stay with babysitters from time to time because my dad worked overnights in the transportation industry. I remember having a friend—if I remember correctly, her name was JoBell. She was the daughter of one of my mother's work colleagues, and I would go to her house after school and wait for my mother to pick me up.

One day, my mother styled my hair in two braided ponytails—one at the top and one at the bottom—with barrettes and hair bows. When you've been told that your hair is so bad and unmanageable, you don't have an appreciation for it. I didn't care if my hair was short or long, and that was a dangerous combination for a rambunctious eight-year-old. I bet you can imagine what happened next.

JoBell found a pair of scissors, and I can't remember if she dared me or if I came up with the bright idea. But I took those scissors and cut an inch off the top and bottom ponytail. Holding the scissors and two inches of hair in my hands, I thought it was so cool. I was excited to show my mom how I cut my hair.

When it was time to pick me up, I ran downstairs to share my accomplishment! To my surprise, my mom did not share my same excitement. She was shocked. "How did you get those scissors?" she asked me. I shared how we had come up with the bright idea to cut our hair together. Grabbing me by my arm, she quickly ushered me to the car out of frustration. My mother lectured me the whole car ride home. That was my first real lesson on loving my hair—I unfortunately had to learn the hard way.

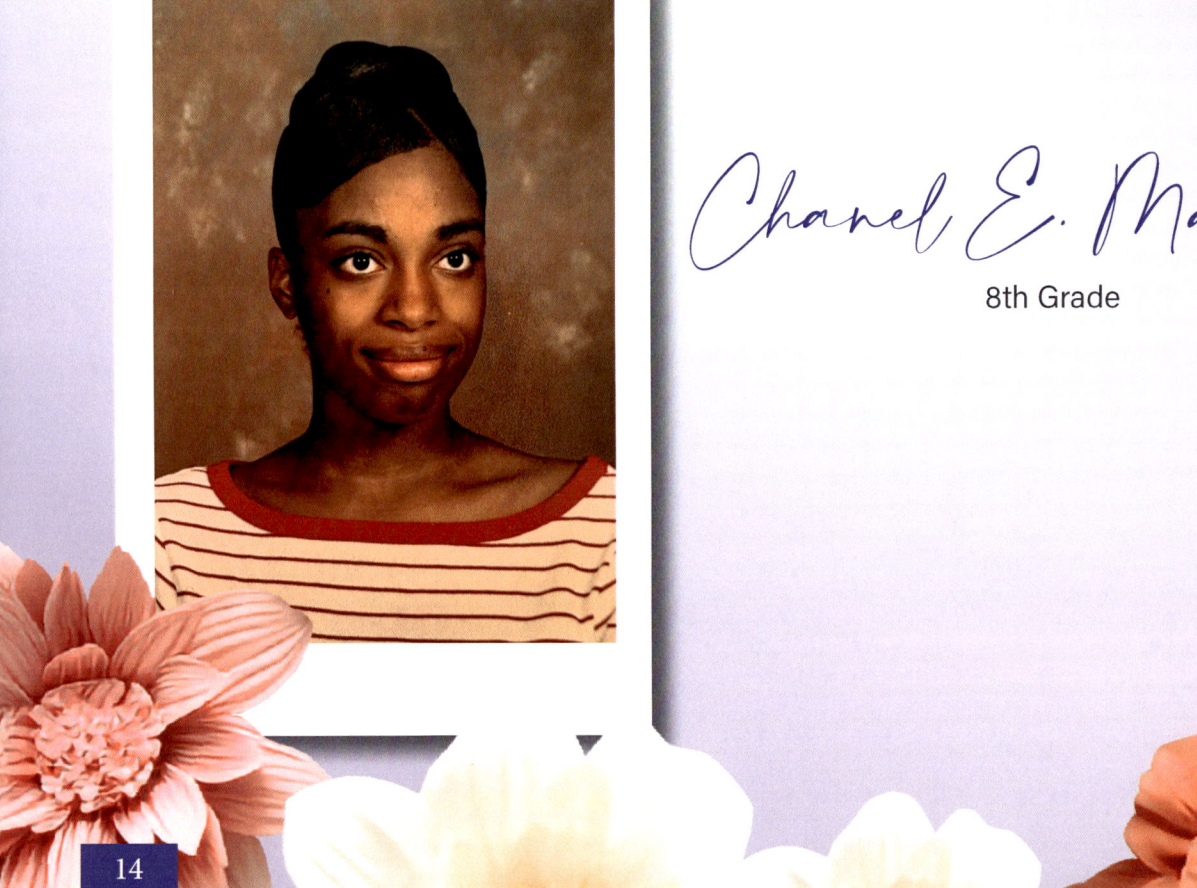

Chanel E. Martin

8th Grade

MORGAN MAKAIL

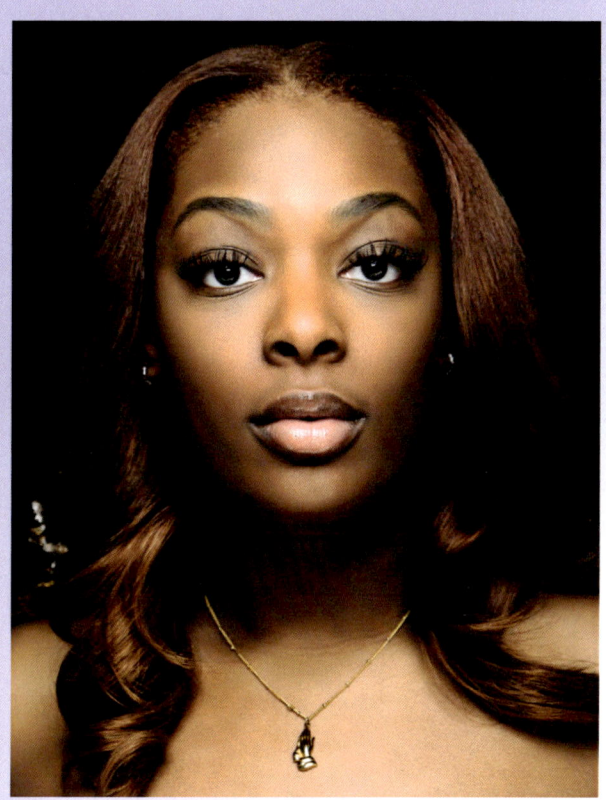

SOCIAL MEDIA HANDLE:

@morgan.makail

ABOUT MORGAN:

Morgan Makail is a life coach, author, and content creator who is passionate about helping women heal from trauma, grow in faith, and walk in purpose. As the founder of WarriHERs, she empowers women to break generational cycles and build confidence. When she's not coaching, Morgan enjoys being in the kitchen, creating new recipes, and baking sourdough.

WHY DO YOU LOVE YOUR HAIR?

"I love my hair for its versatility. Growing up, I once saw my kinky coils as a hassle, never realizing they were a beautiful crown."

FAVORITE BEAUTY OR HAIR HACK:

DRINK your water with lemon! Your skin and waist will thank you later.

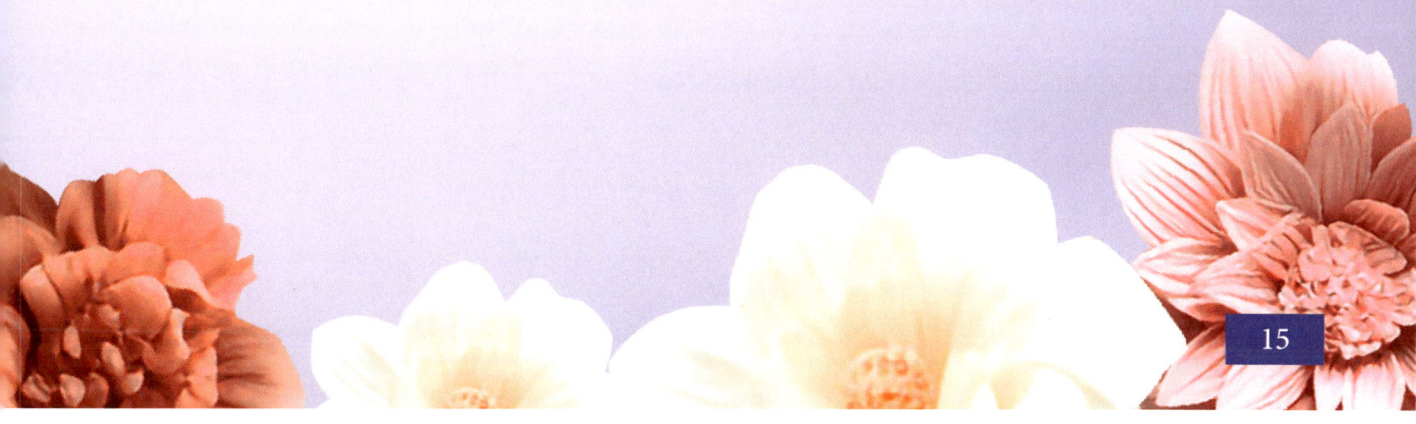

ILEISHA HONEYCUTT

SOCIAL MEDIA HANDLE:

@honeycutt___

ABOUT ILEISHA:

Ileisha Honeycutt is a beauty and fashion creative with over a decade of experience in styling, wigs, and content creation. As a wig influencer and stylist, she helps women feel confident with effortless, on-trend looks. Her background spans bridal beauty, personal styling, and social media, bringing a fresh and relatable approach to the industry. Passionate about storytelling and aesthetics, Ileisha creates engaging beauty content that resonates with today's modern audience.

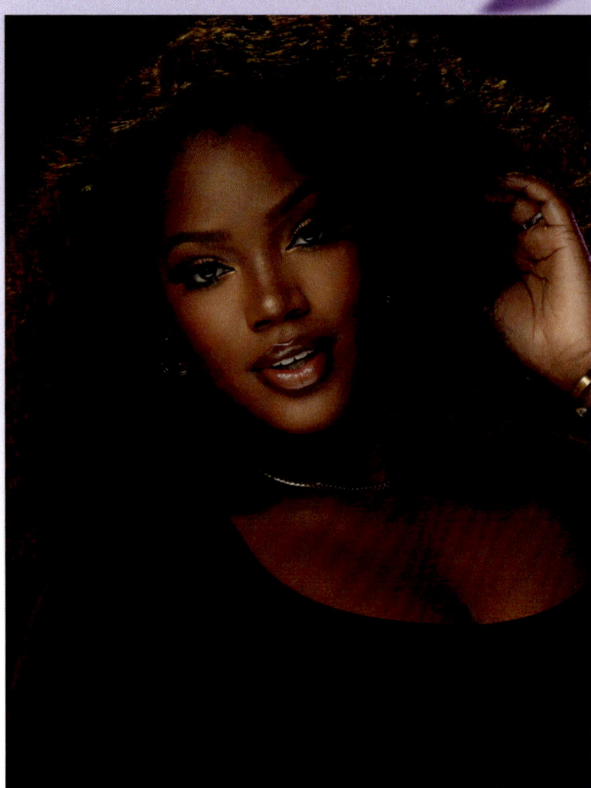

WHY DO YOU LOVE YOUR HAIR?

"My hair is my art—every style tells a story, and every look is a vibe."

FAVORITE BEAUTY OR HAIR HACK:

Always let your wig or extensions air dry for a more natural look and longer-lasting wear.

TE'ETTA RUTH

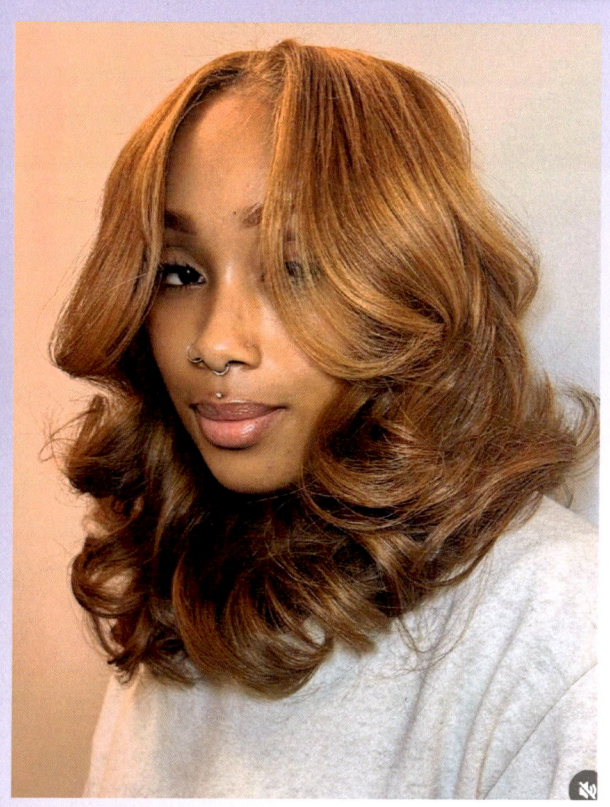

SOCIAL MEDIA HANDLE:

Instagram: @transformingwithtee_
TikTok: @transformingwithtee

ABOUT TE'ETTA:

Te'Etta Ruth is a lifestyle content creator with a passion for faith, home décor, beauty, and wellness. Through her content, she inspires others to live life fully while sharing her own journey in creativity, self-care, and personal growth. With a blend of style, inspiration, and authenticity, Te'Etta invites her audience into every part of her world, encouraging them to embrace intentional living with grace and confidence.

WHY DO YOU LOVE YOUR HAIR?

I love my hair because of its incredible versatility! I've worn it long, short, colored, and in countless styles, each reflecting a different part of me. As a Black woman, I love how our hair allows us to express ourselves in so many beautiful and unique ways.

FAVORITE BEAUTY OR HAIR HACK:

My go-to beauty tip for breakouts is using liquid eyeliner to turn blemishes into beauty marks. It's a simple trick that adds a touch of elegance while seamlessly blending imperfections into your look!

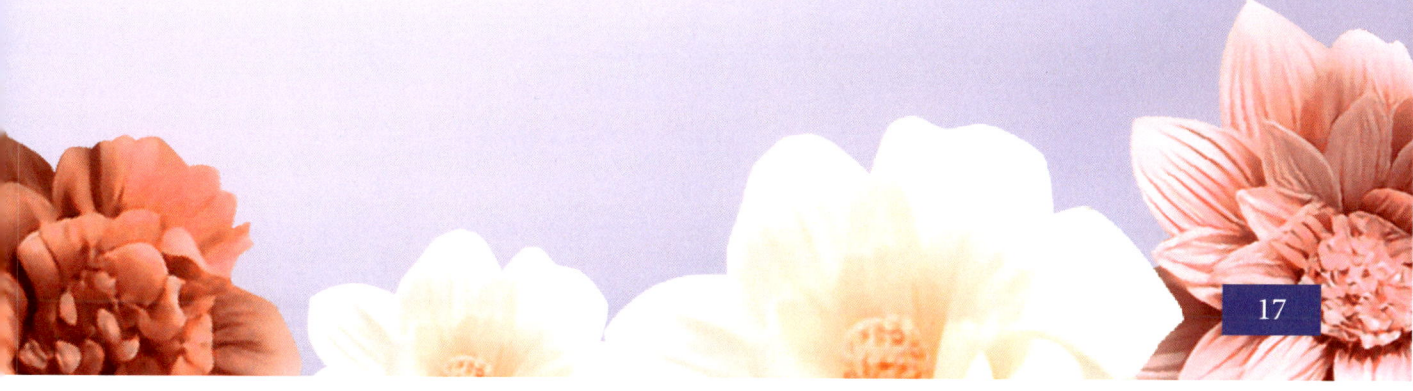

MY DOLL BEAUTY SALON

My fascination with hair and beauty started at a young age. One day, my mother was away at work, and we had an important function to attend that evening. We had one issue: my hair needed to be washed. My dad accepted the charge to wash and style my hair. He sat me over the sink and washed my hair, then proceeded to blow-dry it. Afterward, he put my hair in five messy braids. I rushed to the bathroom, looked in the mirror, and was confused and disappointed. My hair didn't look anything like when my mother styled it. Thankfully, my mother got home in enough time to put my hair in a poofy ponytail. It was at that moment I decided to learn how to do my hair.

I was around eight years old, didn't have anyone to practice on, and decided that my dolls would be my subjects. I had a bunch of Cabbage Patch dolls and a whole host of Barbies. I started with the Barbie dolls, teaching myself how to braid their hair in individual braids. I next experimented with cutting, deciding what styles I wanted to recreate. Searching the Hype Hair magazines, I attempted to recreate the eccentric styles of the 90s.

After I pretty much destroyed all my Barbie dolls' hair, I moved on to the Cabbage Patch dolls! I was going to learn how to cornrow. I asked my mother to show me how to do it. I watched as she grabbed the pieces of hair and how her wrists moved methodically. I memorized the movements—grab one piece of hair, split it into three parts, over, under, over, under, grab another piece of hair, and repeat.

For a whole week, I practiced the movements. Then, finally, I connected a few loose braids on my doll! Bursting with excitement, I rushed to the living room to share my achievement. I could officially braid! That skill would carry me through college and help me with my little girls.

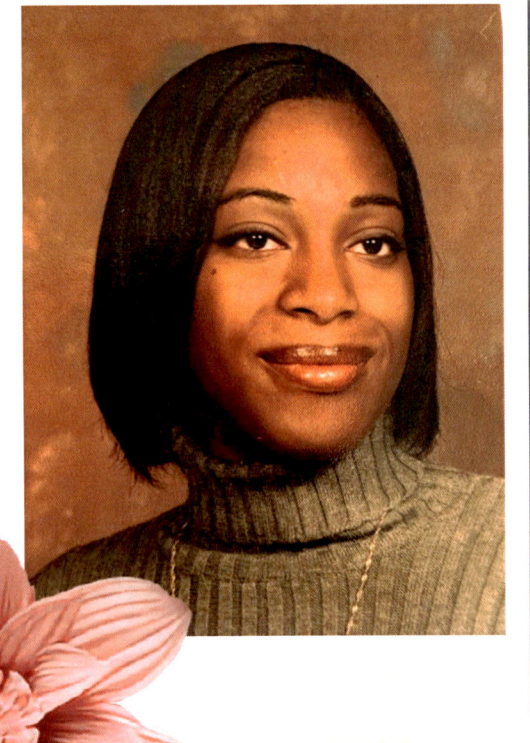

Chanel E. Martin

10th Grade

DR. SHANNETTE BONE

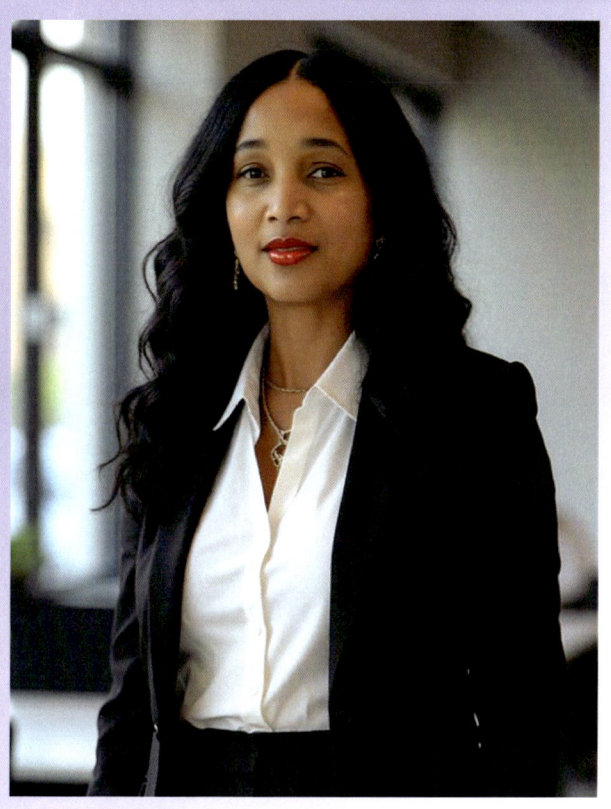

SOCIAL MEDIA HANDLE:

Instagram: @DrShannette Bone
TikTok: @drshannettebone5
YouTube: Dr Shannette Bone
Facebook: DrShannetteBone

ABOUT SHANNETTE:

Dr. Shannette Bone is a woman of integrity and strong character—a true pillar in her community. As a dedicated community advocate, she works tirelessly to support change in areas such as voting rights and gun violence prevention. A proud single mother of four and grandmother of four, Dr. Bone leads with both compassion and conviction. She is the founder of her own nonprofit organization and is deeply committed to empowering, uplifting, and supporting women. Her mission is to be the change she wants to see—not just in her community but across the nation.

WHY DO YOU LOVE YOUR HAIR?

"I love my hair because it matches my personality, my aura. It resonates with me where this is my long hair with a short hair or whether it's braids."

FAVORITE BEAUTY OR HAIR HACK:

My favorite beauty is either you can wear your natural hair or me I love wearing braids so either one I'm comfortable just being able to be comfortable in your own skin either way.

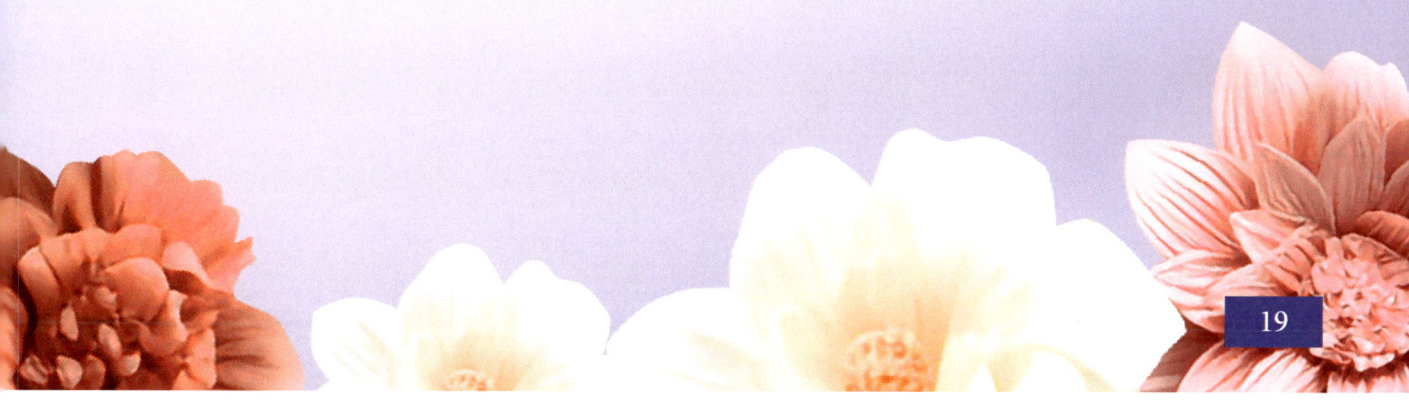

SILVER MORAN-STEWART

SOCIAL MEDIA HANDLE:

Instagram: @_silvermonique
TikTok: It's Silver Monique
YouTube: It's Silver Monique

ABOUT SILVER:

Silver Moran-Stewart is a passionate digital content creator specializing in hair design, hair care, fashion, and education. Known for her engaging videos and educational tutorials, Silver combines authenticity and creativity to deliver content that both inspires and informs. Her work reflects a commitment to producing high-quality, visually appealing content that connects with audiences and leaves a lasting impression.

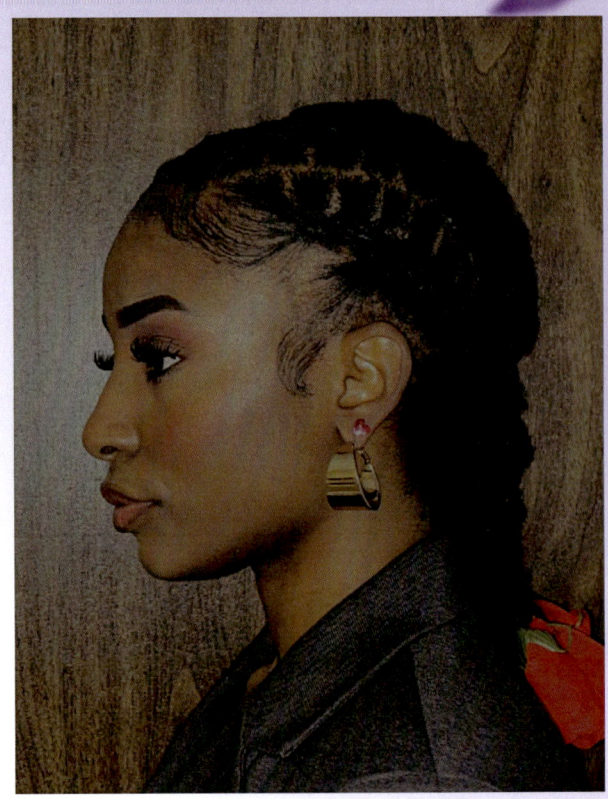

WHY DO YOU LOVE YOUR HAIR?

"I love my hair because it's more than just hair to me; it's a form or art and self-expression."

FAVORITE BEAUTY OR HAIR HACK:

Eat Hair-Healthy Foods – Foods rich in biotin, omega-3s, and protein help locs grow longer and stronger. Hair Tip: Be Mindful of Product Ingredients – Avoid waxes, petroleum, and thick creams that leave residue. Every loc girl knows to wear a satin or silk bonnet to bed to avoid lint but this can also help to prevent dryness while keeping your locs neat.

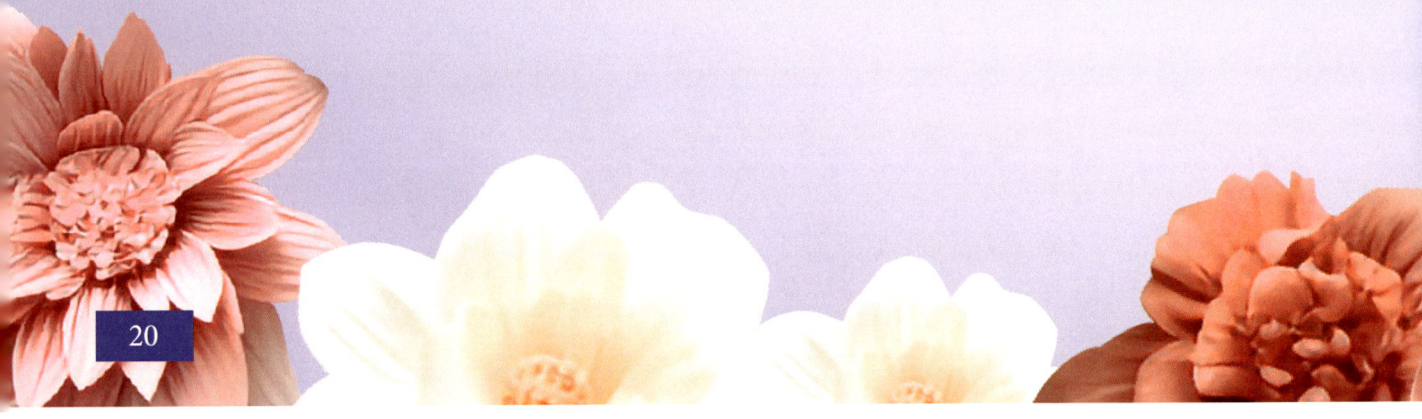

CRYSTAL R. DURHAM

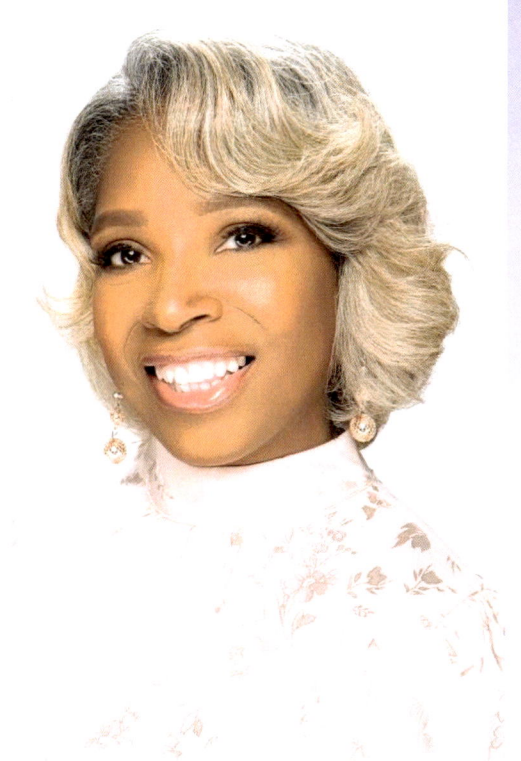

SOCIAL MEDIA HANDLE:

@mrandmrsurham

ABOUT CRYSTAL:

Coach Crystal R. Durham is a nonprofit expert, author, and speaker dedicated to helping women turn their pain into purpose. As a faith-driven leader, she has built successful nonprofits, mentored countless women, and advocated for healing and financial empowerment. With a heart for service and a passion for transformation, she equips others to walk boldly in their God-given calling.

WHY DO YOU LOVE YOUR HAIR?

"I love my hair because it tells a story—one of growth, strength, and authenticity. It's all-natural, a beautiful blend of silver and blonde that shines like wisdom woven into every strand. Healthy, vibrant, and full of life, my hair isn't just an accessory—it's a reflection of who I am. Bold yet soft, strong yet free, it moves with me, complements my personality, and reminds me daily that beauty isn't about fitting in—it's about embracing exactly who God created me to be."

FAVORITE BEAUTY OR HAIR HACK:

Here's a quick hair tip: Be yourself! If you love a press and curl, rock it with confidence. If you love your natural texture, embrace it fully. The key is to shine as your most authentic self!

BOBBING AND BOYS

I was in the 6th grade, and the relaxers had done a number on my hair. I had no choice but to cut it. I remember thinking I was going to get a nice long silky roller wrap. But there was so much breakage after my relaxer touch-up, I had to get a cut. Here I am, 12 years old, and I get my hair cut into a short bob. This bob aged me from 12 to 22. I looked super grown with my new short cut style.

The salon was in the mall, and my mother dropped me off. After the appointment was completed, I decided to walk around the mall and window shop. (This was before I had a cell phone. I'm not exactly sure how I caught up with her later, lol.) While walking in the mall, I was approached by a teenage boy who asked me for my phone number. I'm pretty sure he thought I was at least 15 or 16 with my grown-ish hairstyle. This was also the first time I had ever been approached by a boy I didn't know.

Frozen in fear, I looked at the young man, told him I was only 12, and ran off to find my mom. I found her looking around in Sears (how I knew she'd be there, I don't know) and told her what happened. "Mom, mom, this boy asked me for my number," I frantically shared. My mother looked at me, trying not to laugh, and asked, "Well, what did you tell him?" I explained how I told him I was only 12 and ran. I thought I did the right thing, not understanding that I looked like a grown 22-year-old with my new haircut! My mother explained to me that when you are attractive, young boys will try to get your attention. She also reminded me that I was too young to entertain any of them. Did you ever rock a grown-up hairstyle as a kid?

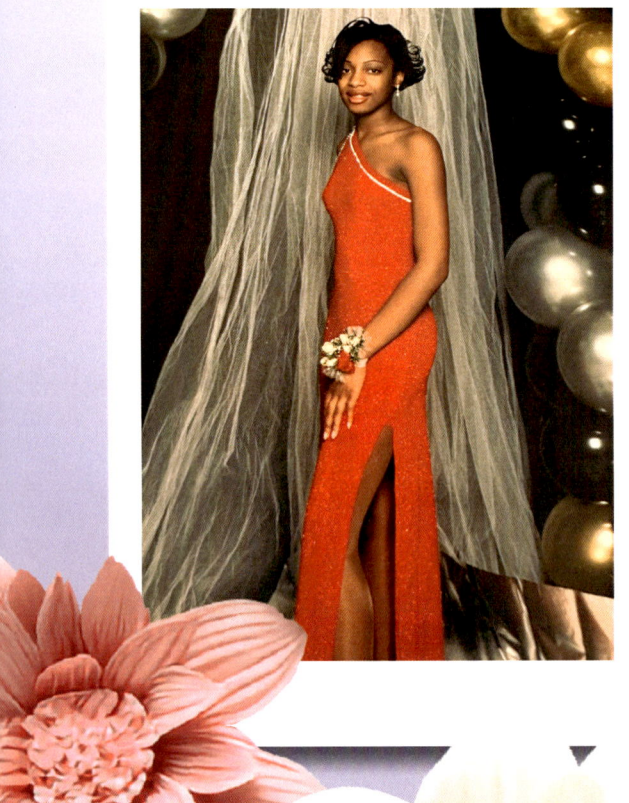

Chanel E. Martin

11th Grade

SARAH NOELSAINT

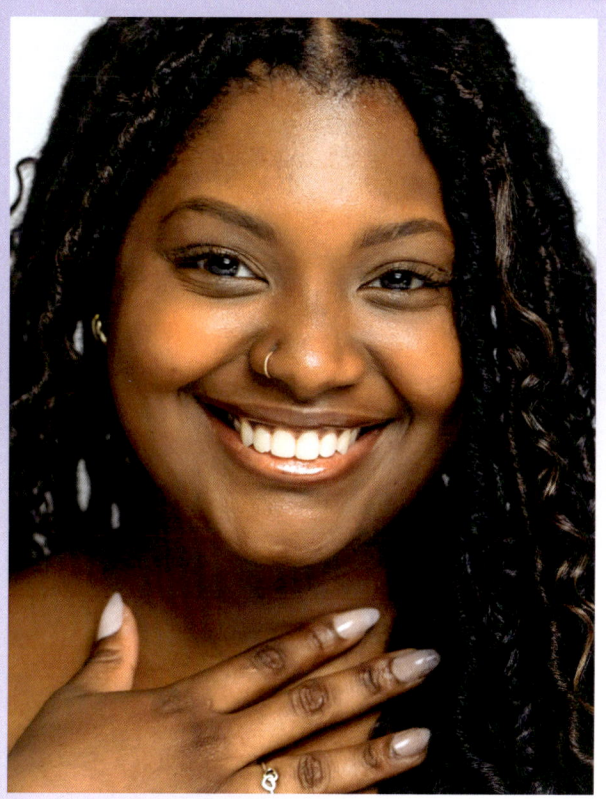

SOCIAL MEDIA HANDLE:

Instagram: @sarahnoelsaint
TikTok: @sarahnoelsaint
Youtube: @sarahnoelsaint

ABOUT SARAH:

Sarah is a model, content creator, and nurse whose heart belongs to creativity. After stepping away from the daily demands of healthcare, she embraced her entrepreneurial spirit and leaned fully into content creation. Known for her authentic voice and artistic expression, Sarah uses her platform to share her journey—offering beauty tips, messages of self-love, and insights on wellness and healing. Through vulnerability and creativity, she inspires others to believe in themselves and pursue the life they were truly meant to live.

WHY DO YOU LOVE YOUR HAIR?

"I love my hair because it's a reflection of my unique beauty. Once I learned to embrace it, it started to grow and love me back. The versatility of my hair reminds me that I'm perfectly made."

FAVORITE BEAUTY OR HAIR HACK:

I swear by eating a balanced diet rich in vitamins and minerals to nourish my hair from the inside out. Staying hydrated and incorporating plenty of fruits, vegetables, and healthy fats has made a noticeable difference in my hair health. Also, I never underestimate the power of sleep protection—using a satin or silk scarf or pillowcase helps prevent breakage and keeps my hair looking smooth, moisturized in the morning!

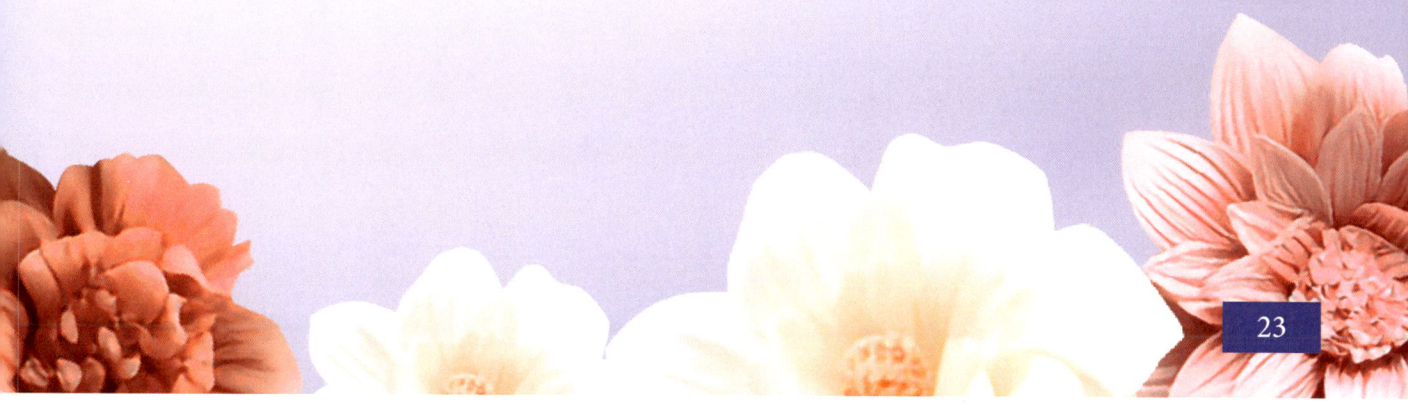

CREE GRIER

SOCIAL MEDIA HANDLE:

@cree8ion

ABOUT CREE:

Cree Grier is a vibrant and influential woman known for her love of beauty, fashion, and giving back. With a bubbly personality and a heart for supporting others, Cree uses her platform to uplift, inspire, and lead by example. Her presence is a blend of style, substance, and service—making a lasting impact both online and in her community.

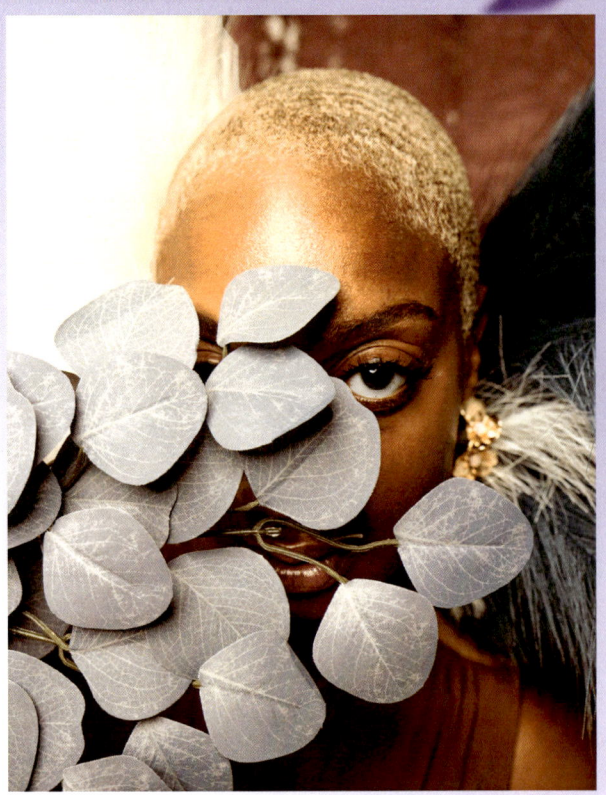

WHY DO YOU LOVE YOUR HAIR?

"I love my hair because it's short, beautiful and it's me! Everyone can't do this style, and I embrace it."

FAVORITE BEAUTY OR HAIR HACK:

You can do anything you want to do if only you try it!

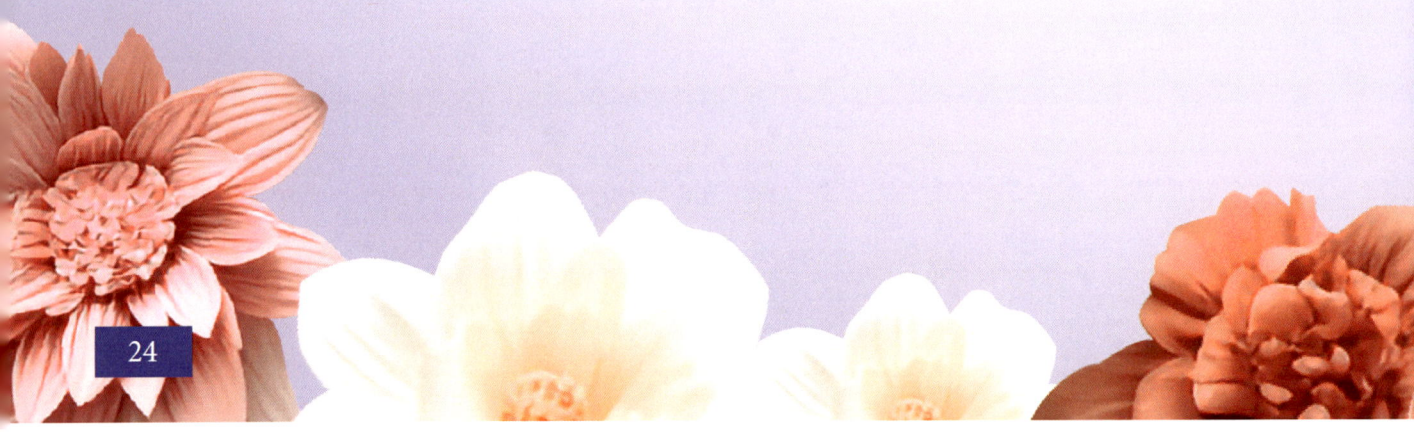

DEJAH JANAE

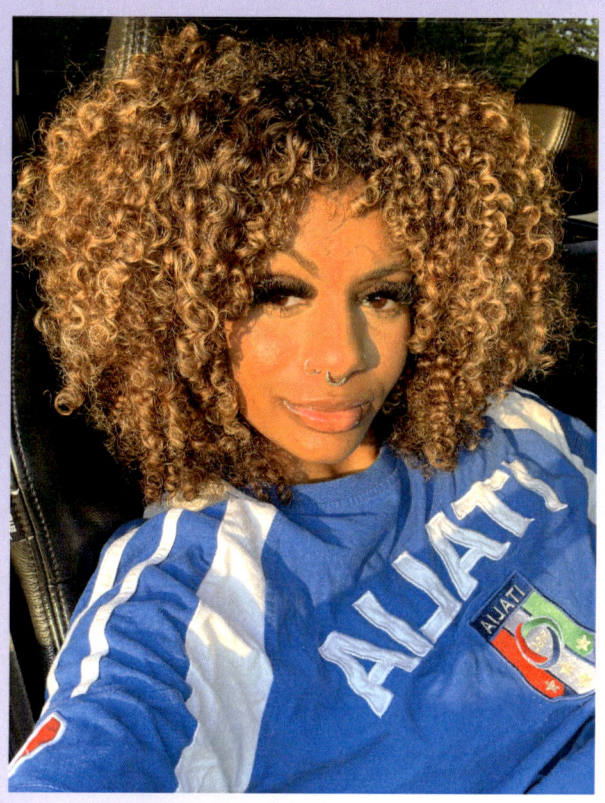

SOCIAL MEDIA HANDLE:

Instagram: @dejahjanae_
TikTok: @dejahjanae

ABOUT DEJAH:

Dejah Janae is a creative entrepreneur, photographer, and digital storyteller with a passion for beauty, wellness, lifestyle, and travel. Her work is rooted in representation, advocacy, and helping others embrace their confidence. Through content creation, brand strategy, and community-building, Dejah empowers others—especially women and people of color—to take up space and own their narratives. At the heart of it all is her faith; Dejah uses her platform to reflect God's love, uplift others, and encourage them to walk boldly in their purpose.

WHY DO YOU LOVE YOUR HAIR?

"I love my hair because it's a reflection of my journey—growth, strength, and self-love. Just like me, my curls have evolved, matured, and embraced their natural beauty. We all go through phases of learning to love our hair, and for me, it was God's gift that I've grown to cherish. It's a symbol of confidence, versatility, and the healthy, loving relationship I've built with myself."

FAVORITE BEAUTY OR HAIR HACK:

Style your curls while they're dripping wet for the best definition! One of my favorite tricks is putting my wash-and-go curls into six braids while I do my makeup. Then, I take them out while they're still wet for a heatless stretch and a perfect mix of defined curls and a braid-out look—all in one!

KOOL-AID COLOR

One day in middle school (7th grade to be exact), I was admiring my friend's bright red highlights in her hair. We were around the same age, and I couldn't believe her parents let her color her hair. I boldly asked her if that was the case. She replied, "No, I dyed my hair with Kool-Aid—the red pack." She got my wheels turning in my head! I knew we had Kool-Aid at home, and I couldn't wait to try it.

I got off the bus and headed straight to the kitchen in search of red Kool-Aid. We didn't have red, but I found pink lemonade. Determined to try it, I followed the instructions she gave me: open the packet, add a little bit of water, pour it on the part of your hair that you want to color, and let it sit. I followed the instructions, and in 15 minutes, I had a streak of pinkish-brown hair on my bangs! "It worked, it worked," I thought to myself. The big test was whether my mom would notice. I anxiously waited for her to come home from work. I was prepared for anything. However, to my surprise, either she didn't notice or she just let me express myself. Either way, it was a win for me!

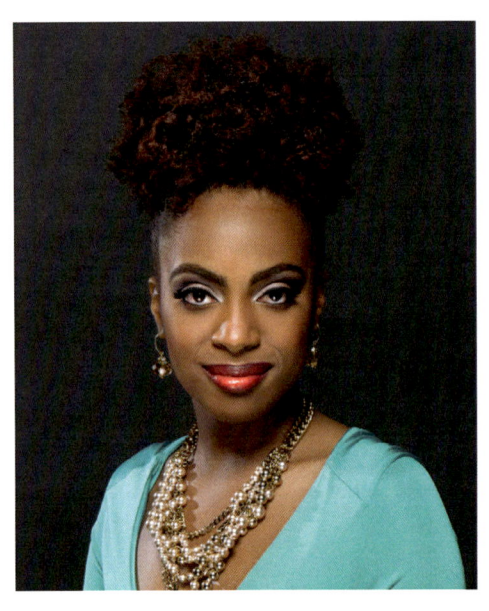

Chanel E. Martin
2013

BARBARA MUKONYO

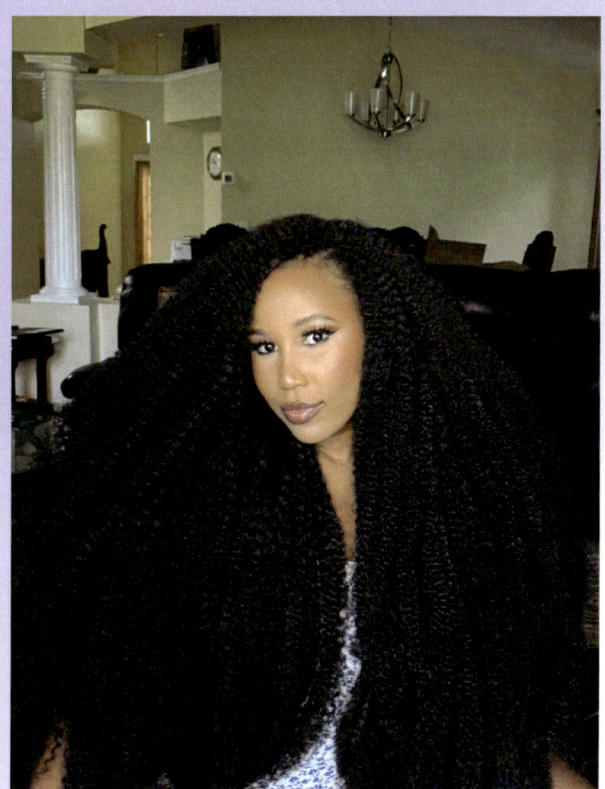

SOCIAL MEDIA HANDLE:

Instagram: @mkn_barbara
TikTok: @bmukonyo

ABOUT BARBARA:

Barbara Mukonyo is a passionate hair content creator based in Orlando, FL, dedicated to teaching girls how to create quick and effective protective styles. Motivated by the gaps in customer service and rising costs in the hair care industry, Barbara uses her platform to offer practical, accessible solutions. In addition to her hair tutorials, she enjoys sharing travel content, combining her love for creativity and exploration to connect with her audience in meaningful ways.

WHY DO YOU LOVE YOUR HAIR?

"Life is too short to have boring hair."

FAVORITE BEAUTY OR HAIR HACK:

I love to swoop my hair in a quick bun while adding Afro kinky extensions, which mimic my hair texture.

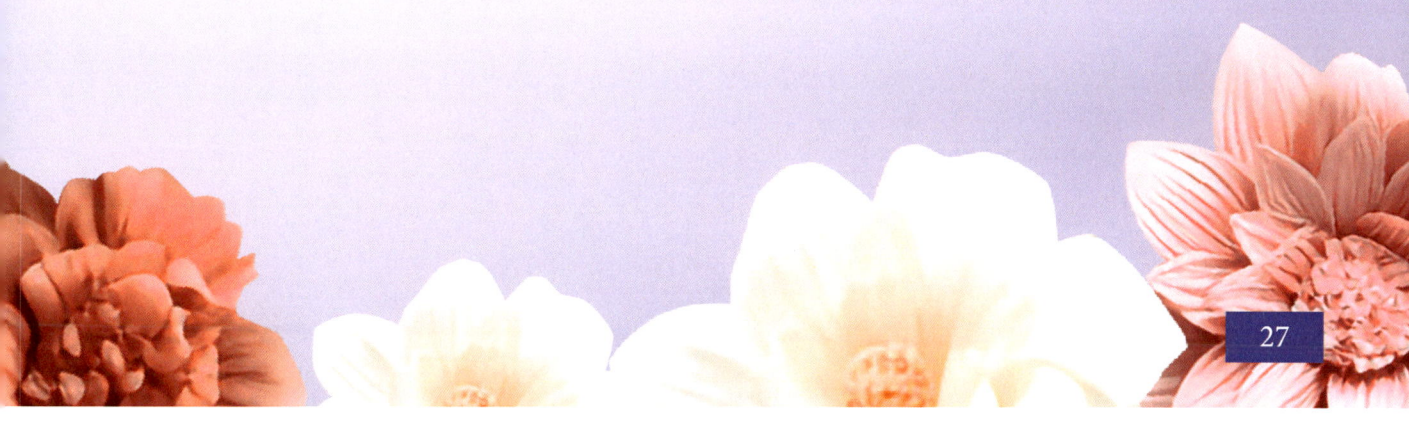

DESTINY THOMAS

SOCIAL MEDIA HANDLE:

@realizing_destiny

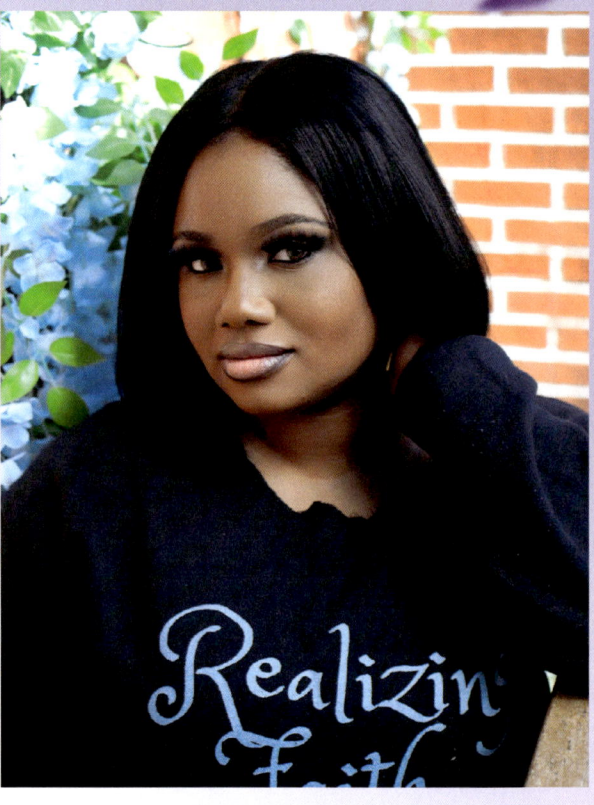

ABOUT DESTINY:

Destiny Thomas, widely known as The Prayerpist®, helps high achievers confidently hear the voice of God so they can gain clarity, heal internally, and avoid self-sabotage during seasons of elevation. She guides clients through a proven 6-step journaling process called Prayerpy®, offering support through one-on-one sessions, her group program Purpose Filled Prayer®, and the Prayerpy Bootcamp.

Destiny is a three-time published author, motivational speaker, and passionate advocate for women battling infertility. She also hosts the annual Prophetic Reloaded Conference and an international retreat, all rooted in her mission to empower others through faith, healing, and purpose.

WHY DO YOU LOVE YOUR HAIR?

"I love my hair because it always reminds me of just how much God loves and cares for me and of the scripture Luke 12:7 Indeed, the very hairs of your head are all numbered. Don't be afraid; you are worth more than many sparrows."

FAVORITE BEAUTY OR HAIR HACK:
Girl, stop carrying all that dead weight, and get those ends trimmed regularly!

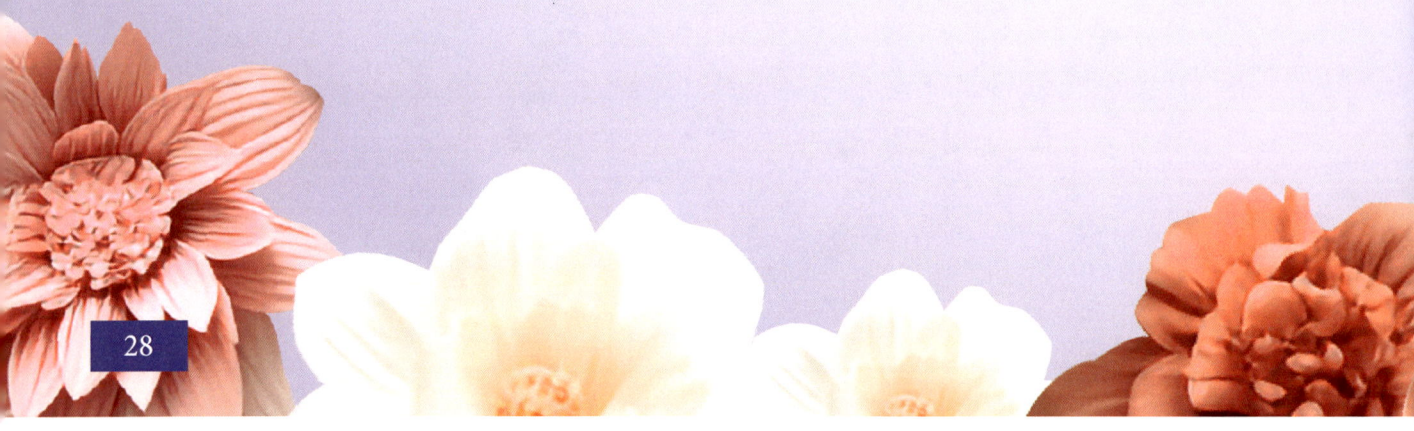

CHRISTAL JORDAN JENNINGS
LENOX & PARKER EDITOR-IN-CHIEF

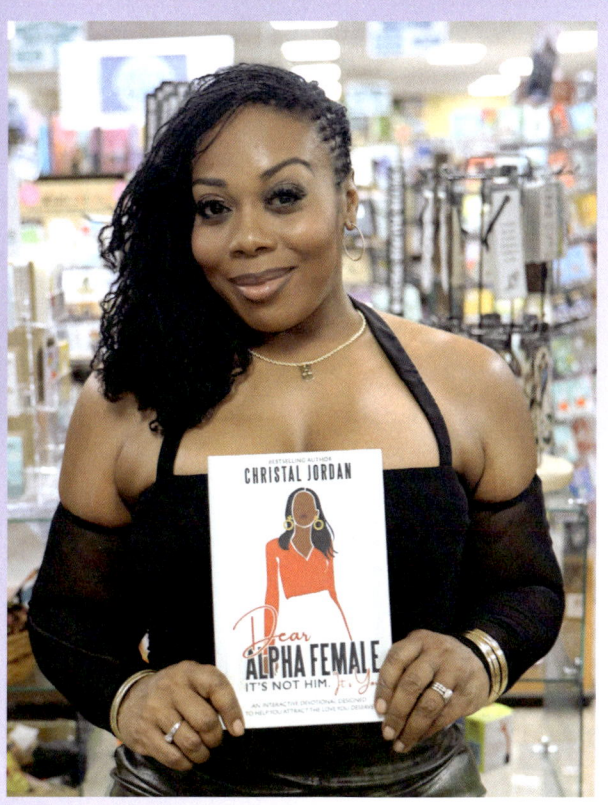

SOCIAL MEDIA HANDLE:

Instagram: @therealchristaljordan,
TikTok: @christaldaniellej,
Youtube: @fromchristalxo

ABOUT CHRISTAL:

Christal Jordan Jennings is an award-winning author and journalist known for her compelling storytelling and insightful features. She currently serves as Editor-in-Chief of Lenox & Parker magazine and is a senior features writer for Collider. Outside of her work in media, Christal is an avid equestrienne who enjoys competing in amateur shows with her quarter horse, Zuri.

WHY DO YOU LOVE YOUR HAIR?

"I recently loc'd my hair after years of wearing weaves, extensions, and wigs. Although I love my hair in any state, in this stage of my life, I'm embracing my authentic self and love the flexibility of microlocs."

FAVORITE BEAUTY OR HAIR HACK:

Moisture is the key to looking young and staying healthy! I moisturize my skin twice a day, and I moisturize my scalp three times a week with rose water.

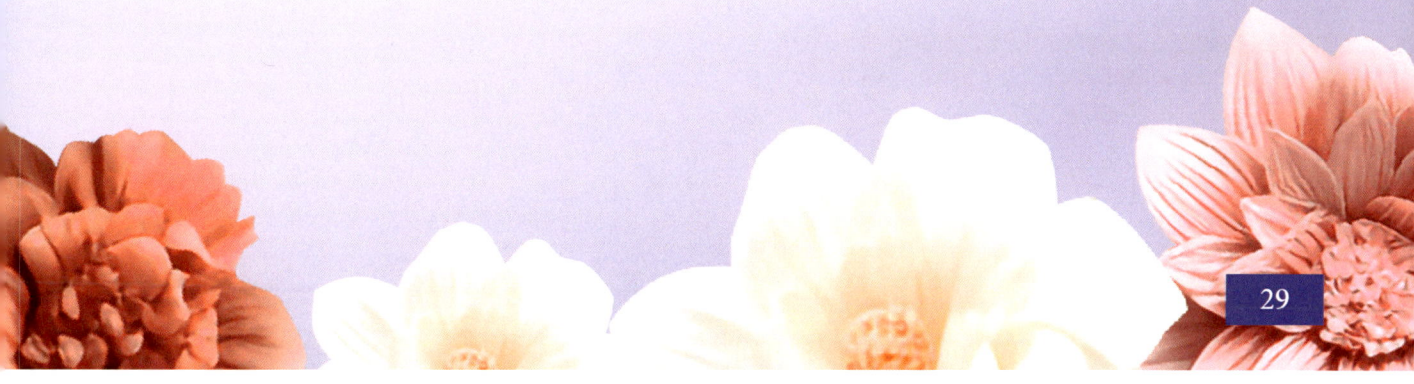

MICRO BRAIDS AND MICROWAVES

Growing up in a single-parent household with my mom working hard for the money, I was determined to learn how to do my hair by myself! I spent hours in the mirror, sneaking my mother's hair products, attempting to style my hair. When I went to the salon, I would study the stylists and memorize the products and steps they took to achieve certain styles.

In the late 90s, skinny crochet braids were extremely popular. One summer at my grandmother's house, I asked my cousin if I could experiment on her. To my surprise, she said yes. That summer, I styled her and my hair in those crinkly, skinny micro crochet braids (y'all remember those, lol).

I washed, braided, and crocheted the hair in the hallway of my grandmother's house. She had a huge mirror that hung on the wall, and it was the perfect faux salon setup. I had done such a great job that my aunt invited me to come stay in Mississippi with my other cousins for a month to style their hair as well. I was so excited to get other heads I could experiment on.

That summer, I perfected my crochet braid method but also picked up a new skill—microwave ponytails. If you forgot about microwave ponies, let me un-jog your memory. You would take a 10-14 inch human hair track bundle, spray it with Pump It Up spray, roll it with rollers, and place it in the microwave for a few minutes. Once completed, you'd have the perfectly curled ponytail. Next, you'd take some Ampro black gel and slick your hair into a high ponytail bun. Finally, you would wrap the weave bundle around your bun and secure each level with bobby pins. And voilà—the perfect ponytail was achieved!

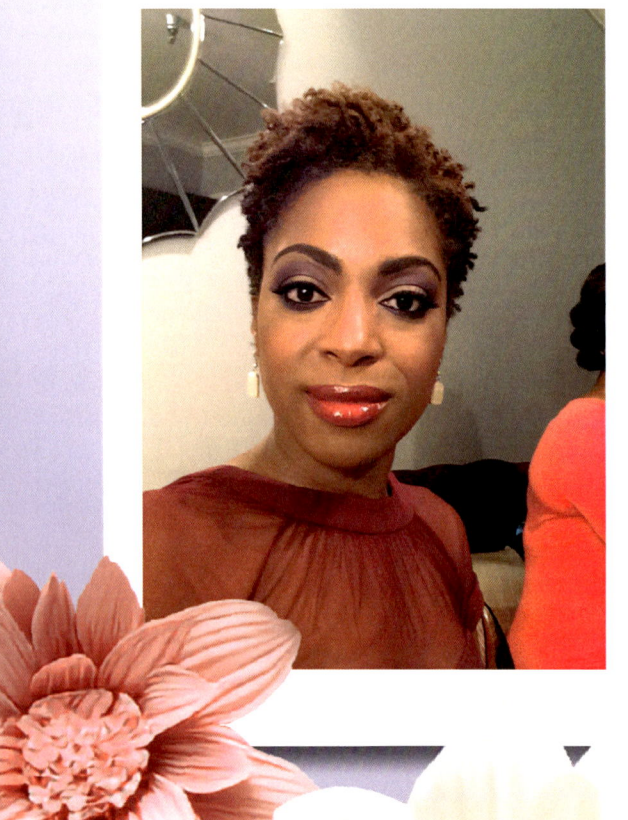

Chanel E. Martin

2015

KENNEDY SIMONE

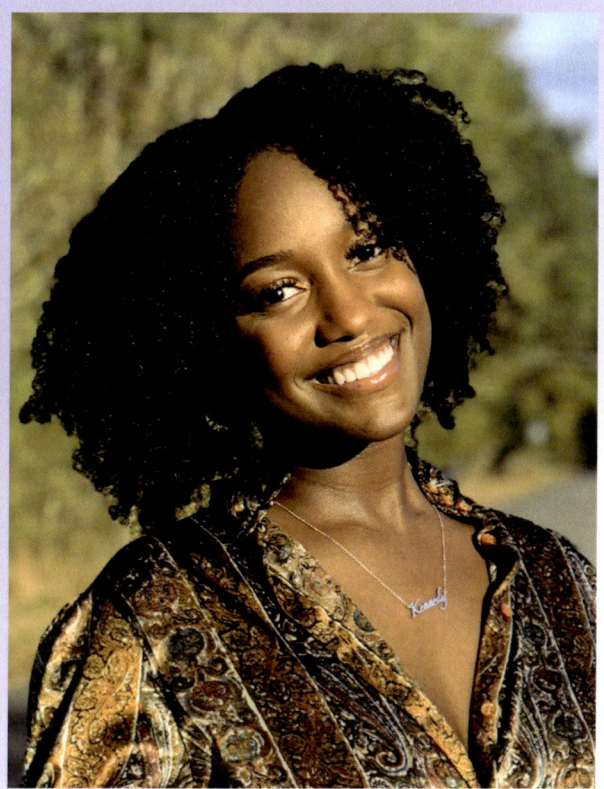

SOCIAL MEDIA HANDLE:

Instagram: @KENNEDYSIMONE
TikTok: @officialkennedysimone
Youtube: @OfficialKennedySimone

ABOUT KENNEDY:

Kennedy Simone is a content creator passionate about self-care, beauty, and inspiring others to embrace their natural confidence. Known for her authentic voice and love for all things hair care, Kennedy shares her personal journey to encourage her audience to feel comfortable and confident in their own skin. On and off the clock, she brings intention and creativity to her content. She's excited to be part of the Her Beauty Regimen community, where she continues to share her passion for natural beauty and self-love.

WHY DO YOU LOVE YOUR HAIR?

"I love my hair because it's imperfectly perfect, just like me—unique, full of character, and a true reflection of who I am!"

FAVORITE BEAUTY OR HAIR HACK:

My favorite hair hack is using a silk scarf, bonnet, or pillowcase to protect my curls overnight. It helps minimize frizz and keeps my hair looking fresh in the morning!

TIFFANY B. LIVINGSTON

SOCIAL MEDIA HANDLE:

@_february4

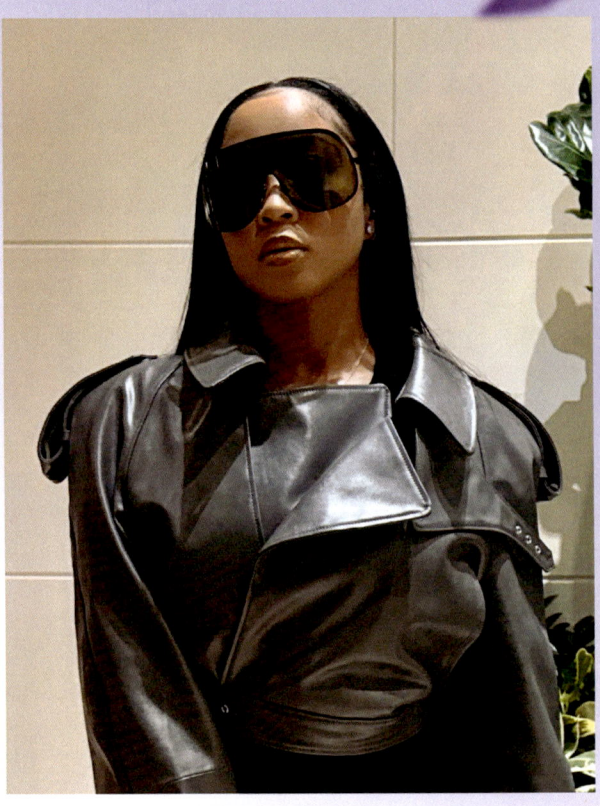

ABOUT TIFFANY:

Tiffany B. Livingston is a Washington, DC native with a deep love for her hometown—no matter how far her travels take her, she always finds her way back. A proud graduate of Hampton University and a member of Alpha Kappa Alpha Sorority, Inc., Tiffany is passionate about beauty, fashion, and wellness. She values quality time with family and friends and is committed to giving back to her community every chance she gets.

WHY DO YOU LOVE YOUR HAIR?

"My hair is a reflection of my personality — wild, free, and always changing."

FAVORITE BEAUTY OR HAIR HACK:
I swear by wrapping my hair at night!

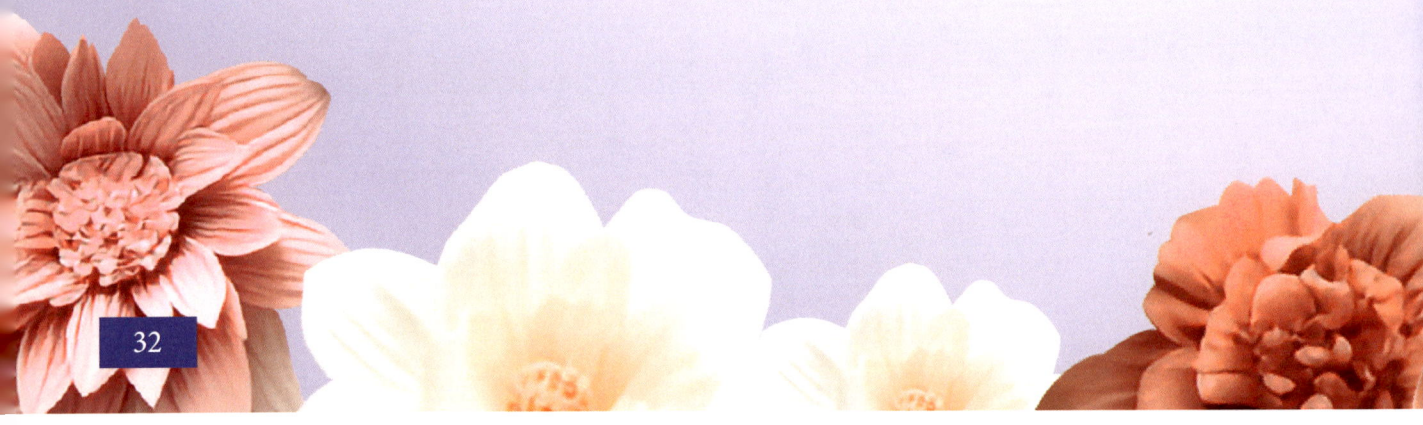

JADE NADAREE

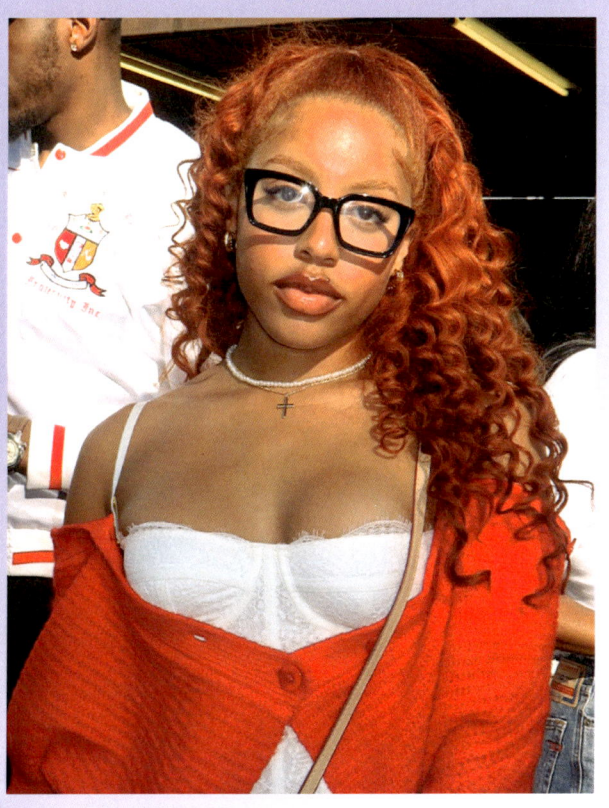

SOCIAL MEDIA HANDLE:

Instagram: @jade_nadaree
TikTok: @jade_nadaree
Youtube: @jadenadaree

ABOUT JADE:

Jade Nadaree is a content creator who shares her journey through post-grad life, focusing on career, beauty, and lifestyle content. Her natural hair journey began in high school when she decided to move away from monthly silk presses that were damaging her hair. Since then, Jade has embraced her curls and learned how to care for them—especially after coloring her hair. She continues to explore new styles and techniques to maintain healthy hair while fully embracing her natural texture and encouraging others to do the same.

WHY DO YOU LOVE YOUR HAIR?

"It grows from my scalp—my beautiful mane, created by God. How could I not love it?"

FAVORITE BEAUTY OR HAIR HACK:

As someone who has struggled with heat-damaged hair, a flexi rod set is my go-to for bringing my curls back to life and achieving the juicy curls I love!

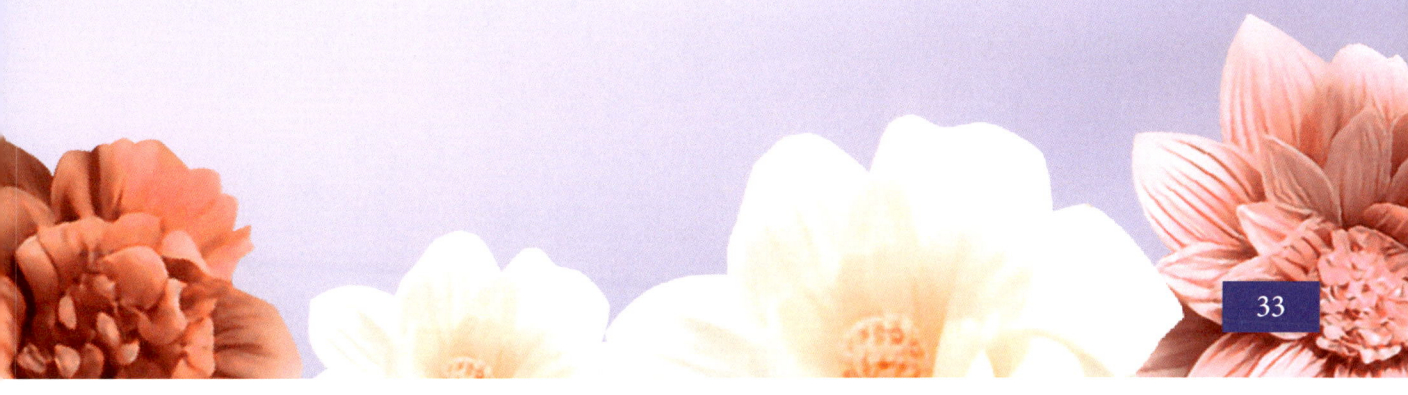

LINDSEY A. WALKER

SOCIAL MEDIA HANDLE:

@lindseyawalker

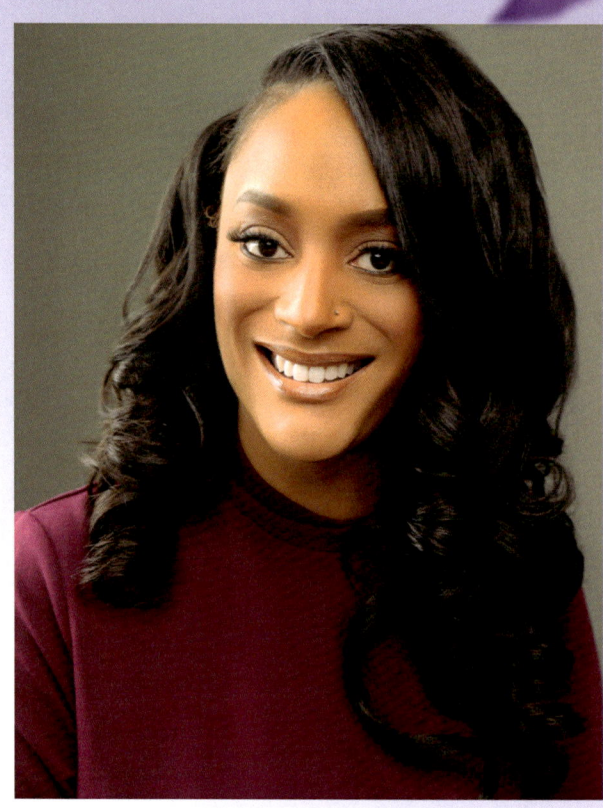

ABOUT LINDSEY:

Lindsey Walker is the founder of Walker + Associates Media Group, a premier publicity agency specializing in securing national media coverage for beauty, beverage, entertainment, and lifestyle brands. With a track record of landing clients in top-tier outlets like Essence, The New York Times, and Forbes, Lindsey is known for her strategic approach to PR that drives real results. As a stage IV cancer survivor and author of Thriving Through The Storm, she is passionate about storytelling that not only amplifies brands but also inspires resilience and impact.

WHY DO YOU LOVE YOUR HAIR?

"My hair is more than just strands—it's a symbol of resilience, growth, and the grace of God. After losing it to six months of chemo, watching it return has given me a new appreciation for the strength within me. Every curl and coil is a reminder that I survived, and I am thriving."

FAVORITE BEAUTY OR HAIR HACK:

Hydration is key! I swear by using Her Beauty Regimen's Refresh oil to keep my hair moisturized and prevent breakage. Also, I sleep with a satin pillowcase at night, which is a game-changer for protecting my hair!

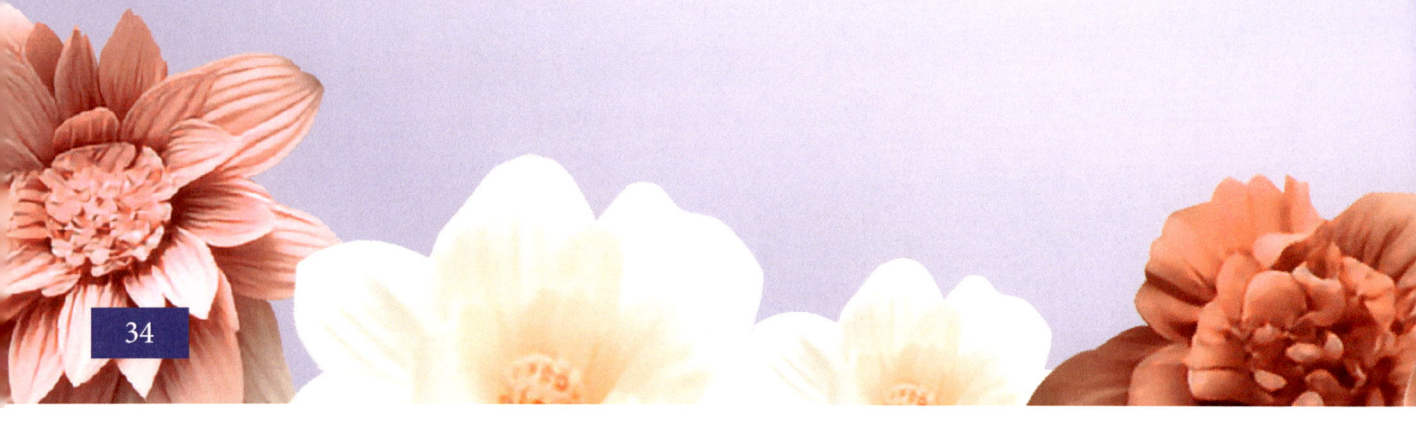

MICRO BRAIDS AND MICROWAVES

Growing up in a single-parent household with my mom working hard for the money, I was determined to learn how to do my hair by myself! I spent hours in the mirror, sneaking my mother's hair products, attempting to style my hair. When I went to the salon, I would study the stylists and memorize the products and steps they took to achieve certain styles.

In the late 90s, skinny crochet braids were extremely popular. One summer at my grandmother's house, I asked my cousin if I could experiment on her. To my surprise, she said yes. That summer, I styled her and my hair in those crinkly, skinny micro crochet braids (y'all remember those, lol).

I washed, braided, and crocheted the hair in the hallway of my grandmother's house. She had a huge mirror that hung on the wall, and it was the perfect faux salon setup. I had done such a great job that my aunt invited me to come stay in Mississippi with my other cousins for a month to style their hair as well. I was so excited to get other heads I could experiment on.

That summer, I perfected my crochet braid method but also picked up a new skill—microwave ponytails. If you forgot about microwave ponies, let me un-jog your memory. You would take a 10-14 inch human hair track bundle, spray it with Pump It Up spray, roll it with rollers, and place it in the microwave for a few minutes. Once completed, you'd have the perfectly curled ponytail. Next, you'd take some Ampro black gel and slick your hair into a high ponytail bun. Finally, you would wrap the weave bundle around your bun and secure each level with bobby pins. And voilà—the perfect ponytail was achieved!

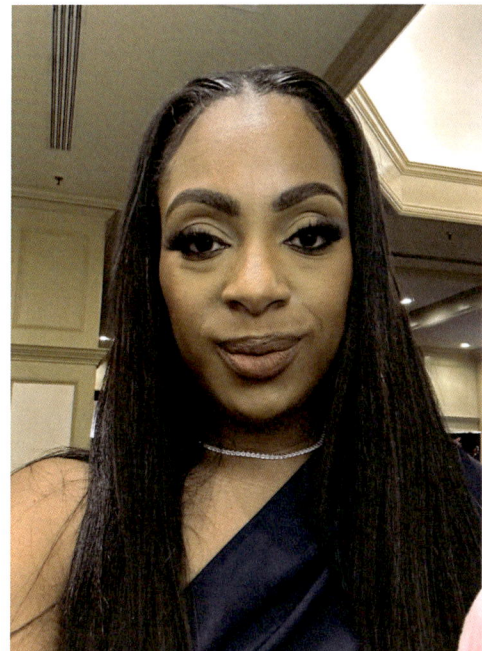

Chanel E. Martin

2014

KARYSE J. GOCOUL

SOCIAL MEDIA HANDLE:

@karysegocoul

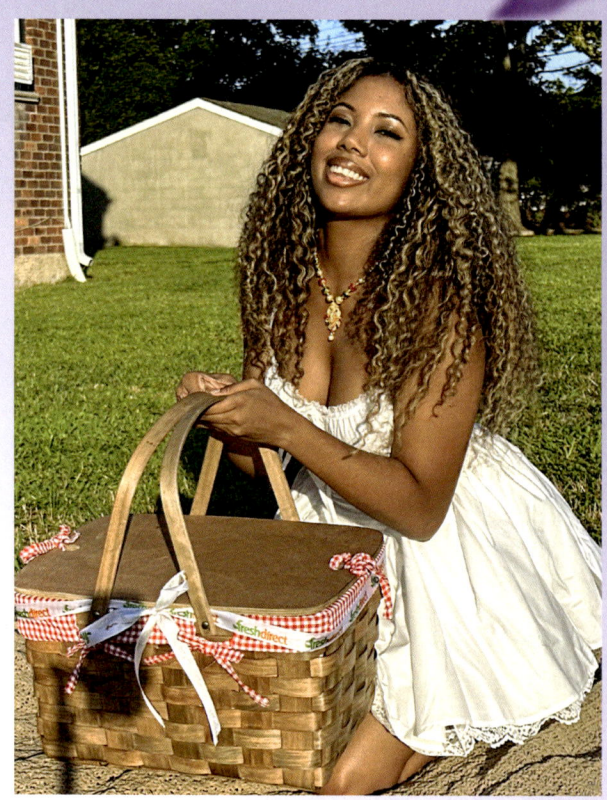

ABOUT KARYSE:

Karyse J. Gocoul is a Content Creator, Journalist, and Model/Actress based in New York. She specializes in travel, lifestyle, hair, fashion, and beauty—bringing a vibrant and polished touch to everything she shares. Karyse is also a proud Miss New York USA 2025 State Finalist, using her platform to inspire and connect with audiences through creativity, confidence, and style.

WHY DO YOU LOVE YOUR HAIR?

"I love my hair because it's big, bold, and unapologetic. It's taken me years to embrace my big, long, mixed texture hair, and I'm happy to have been learning to style and love my hair even more as the years go on."

FAVORITE BEAUTY OR HAIR HACK:
Oiling your scalp while massaging it and also making your own DIY hair treatments!

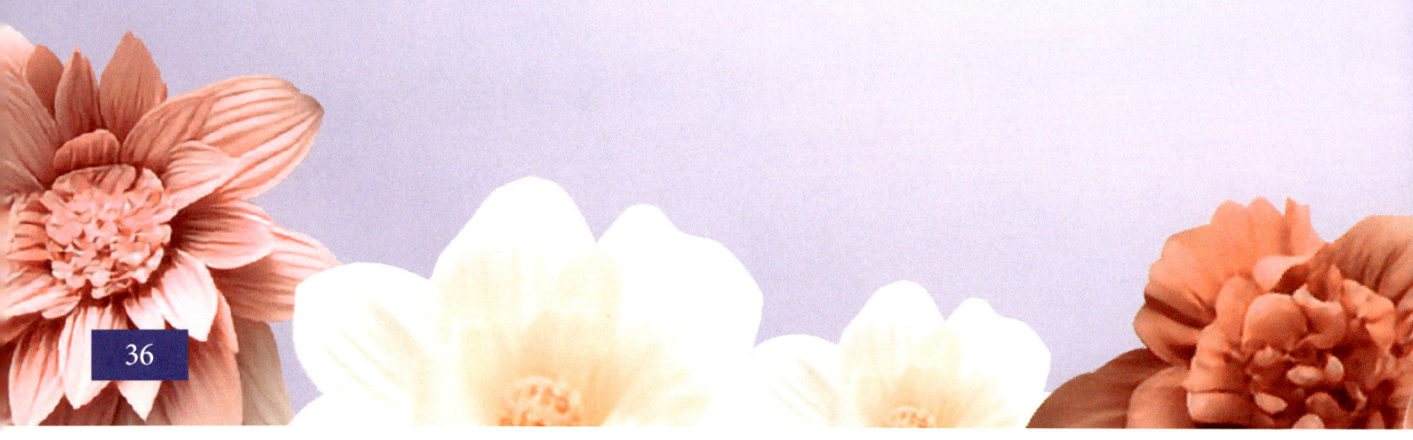

SHIANN GRANEAU

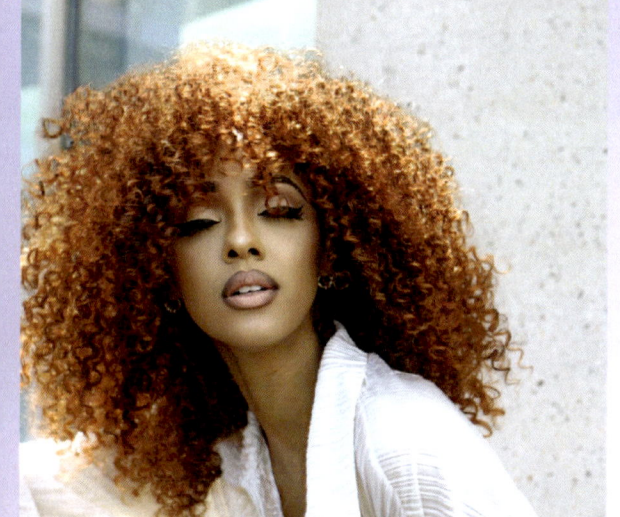

SOCIAL MEDIA HANDLE:

@shiann_graneau

ABOUT SHIANN:

I am of Puerto Rican and West Indian descent (The island of Dominica. I am a digital creator and influencer loving all things beauty, lifestyle, fashion and sports. I am a proud graduate of The University of Central Florida and The University of Miami. I love learning new things and traveling as much as my sky miles will let me!

WHY DO YOU LOVE YOUR HAIR?

"When in doubt, I will always wear my natural hair out!"

FAVORITE BEAUTY OR HAIR HACK:

A good detangling brush and conditioner saves lives.

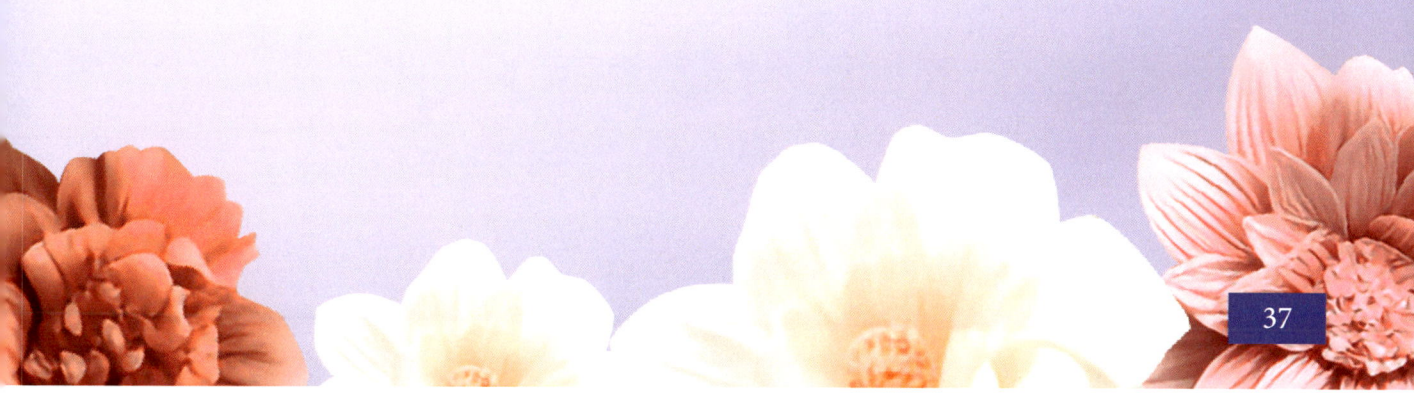

CHANEL E. MARTIN

SOCIAL MEDIA HANDLE:

Instagram: @chanelemartin
TikTok: @chanelemartin
Youtube: @chanelemartin

ABOUT CHANEL:

Chanel E. Martin, Founder of Her Beauty Regimen and the visionary behind this project, is an award-winning serial entrepreneur. Martin is passionate about helping brands build wealth and establish authority via media, books, and entrepreneurship. As a master's degree chemical engineer, Chanel applies a systemic approach to business development and has helped thousands of business owners do the same.

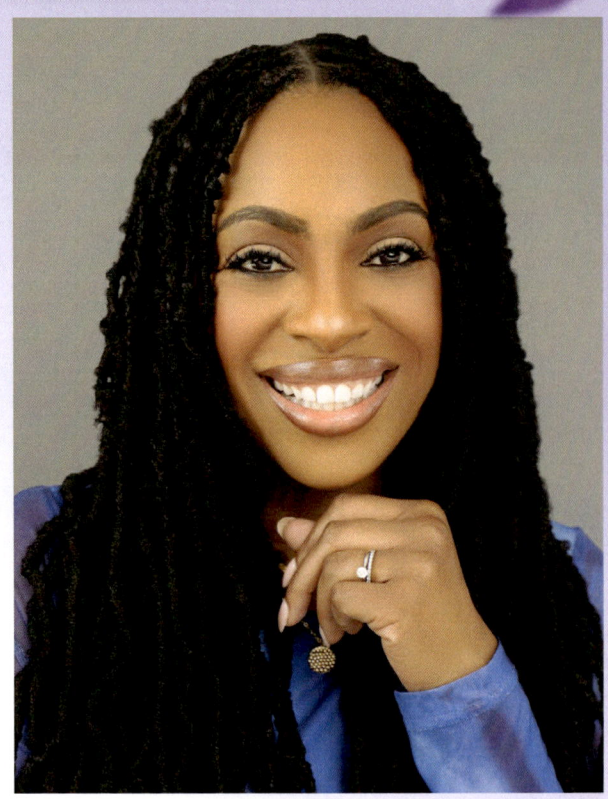

WHY DO YOU LOVE YOUR HAIR?

"I love the versatility of my hair and my willingness to switch it up. You never know what style you are going to get. From wigs to weave, to faux locs, or blow out. I love that I don't have to stick to one look."

FAVORITE BEAUTY OR HAIR HACK:

Of course, I recommend using my Her Beauty Regimen Refreshed Hair & Scalp Growth Oil 3 times a week for stronger, longer hair. But I also love heatless curls. They help protect the integrity of your hair while giving you gorgeous curls.

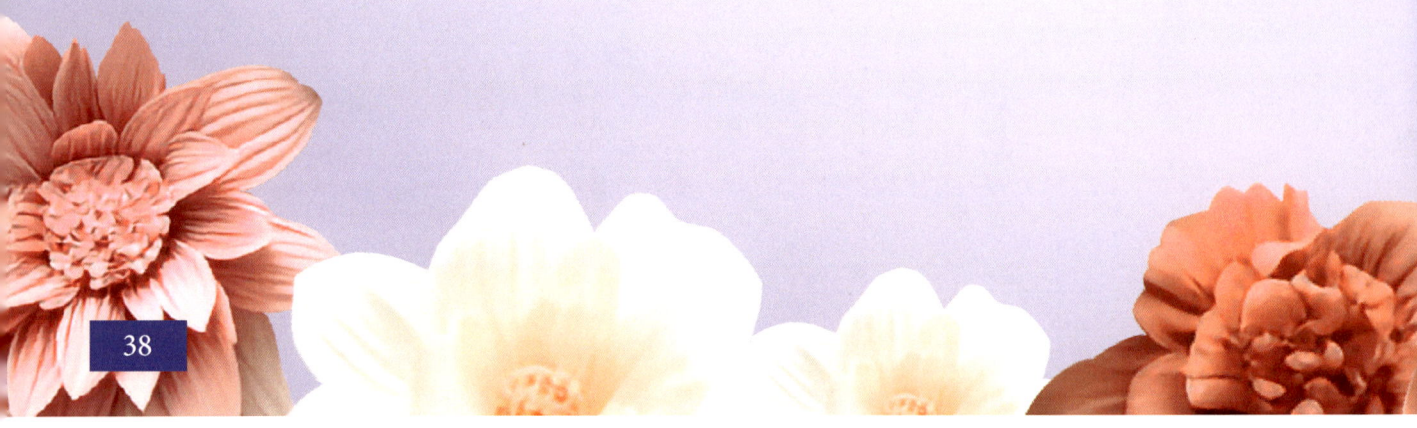

This Lookbook is more than a showcase, it's a love letter to our hair, our stories, and the beauty of showing up as our full selves.

Through the pages of this book, you've read personal reflections from powerful women who are redefining what it means to love their hair. You've seen beauty in every coil, kink, curl, and crown. You've learned about the science, intention, and personal journey behind Refreshed Hair & Scalp Oil—a product born not from hype but from lived experience, research, and a calling to serve women who deserve better.

As a woman who's walked the path of hair loss, healing, and hair care with purpose, I know what it means to want to feel good in your own skin, to want products that honor your journey, not erase it. I'm so proud to share this space with you and the 50 incredible influencers who brought their voices, their confidence, and their truth to this campaign.

Let this be a reminder: You are not alone in your hair journey. There's power in every strand, strength in every story, and beauty in every phase of becoming.

Whether you're starting fresh or thriving in your routine, Her Beauty Regimen is here to support you with products that are backed by science, inspired by real life, and made for women like you.

You can shop Refreshed Hair & Scalp Oil and more at herbeautyregimen.com and join our growing community of beauty lovers and storytellers by following us on social @hbrbrand across all platforms.

We'll be here, cheering you on, helping you grow, and reminding you to love your hair a little more each day.

Chanel E. Martin
Founder, Her Beauty Regimen

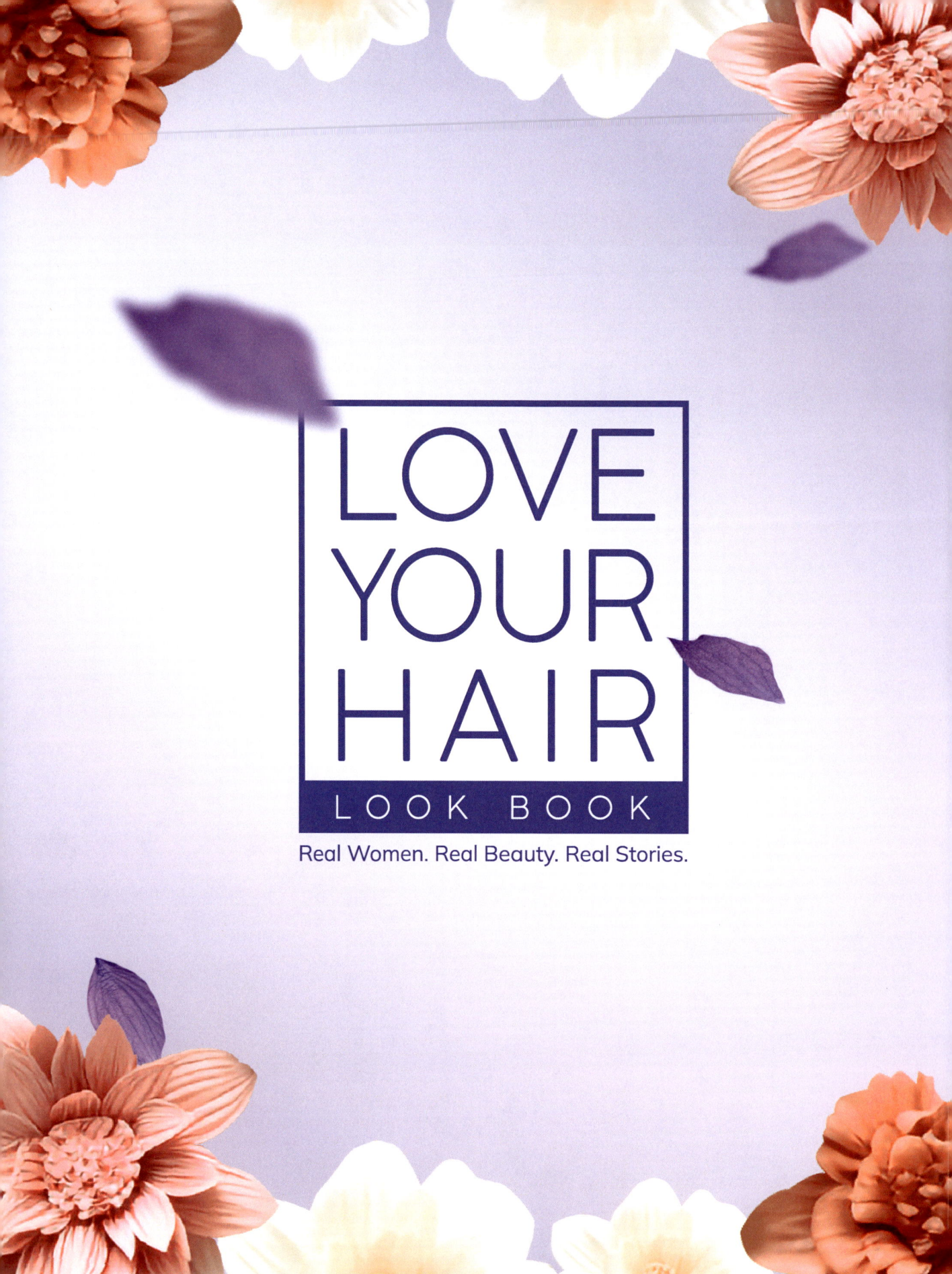

www.ingramcontent.com/pod-product-compliance
Lightning Source LLC
Chambersburg PA
CBRC091205010526
44107CB00021B/1248